Yoga
The Back Pain Cure

YOGA
The Back Pain Cure

The Yoga Therapy Back Care and Low Back Pain Treatment Program

HOWARD VAN ES, E-RYT500 & DR. RICK HARVEY, D.C.

Yoga: The Back Pain Cure
The Yoga Therapy Back Care and Low Back Pain Treatment Program

Howard VanEs, M.A. E-RYT 500 and Dr. Rick Harvey, D.C.

Published by:
BooksOnHealth.net

ISBN: 978-0615986364

Disclaimer: The information and ideas in this book are for educational purposes only. This book is not intended to be a substitute for consulting with an appropriate health care provider. Any changes or additions to your medical care should be discussed with your physician. The authors and publisher disclaim any liability arising directly or indirectly from this book.

Acknowledgements

With deep gratitude, we'd like to thank all of our teachers, patients, and students past, present, and future. Without them this work would not be possible.

We would also acknowledge and thank our yoga model: Suraya Keating

surayasusana@yahoo.com | www.suraya.org

Table of Contents

Introduction

If you're reading this book, chances are very good that that either you or someone you love is experiencing lower back problems. In fact, over 80% of people in the U.S. will have back problems at some point in their lives. That's 240 million people, of which 20% to 30% at any one time will have back problems.

And as anyone with back challenges can attest, back problems are not a lot of fun. Back pain, limited activities, and days missed from work all take their toll physically, financially, and emotionally.

Back problems occur for a variety of reasons including accidents, disease states like arthritis, genetic factors, and lifestyle issues.

One of the big problems with most back care programs is that there have been limited treatment options. Pain medications often just mask problems, allowing further damage to occur because you don't feel the pain. Physical therapy treatment is often limited by what the insurance companies deem necessary, and lastly surgery, a very costly option that is becoming more effective, still often fails.

The good news is that yoga therapy can help relieve your pain while at the same time, improve your flexibility and strength. And because yoga is a practice for the entire mind and body, most people find they sleep better, their mood improves, and they enjoy an enhanced sense of overall well-being.

For over 5000 years, yoga has been helping people find balance in their lives and improve the health of their body, mind, and spirit. Today, yoga's extraordinary popularity is a testament to its profound ability to heal — some 20.4 million people are practicing yoga in the US (according to *Yoga Journal*).

Two pioneers in the application of yoga therapy for back care are Howard VanEs, M.A., E-RYT500 and Dr. Rick Harvey. Howard is a yoga instructor with over 18 years of teaching experience, and Dr. Rick Harvey is a chiropractor with over 36 years of experience. They have worked together to develop a systematic approach for using gentle yoga postures to address lower back care problems. Their program has become so successful that 93% of people with lower back problems who use it either completely heal or significantly reduce pain and regain flexibility.

As you read through this book, you will gain an understanding of the different types of lower back problems, why they occur, what you can do to prevent them and minimize pain and symptoms. In the "first aid" section, you will discover highly effective natural methods for dealing with pain, and, in the lifestyle section, we'll share some tips to keep back problems from becoming a problem in the first place.

In the yoga therapy section of this book, there are two practices. The first is for people who have acute lower back problems. In other words, you are in pain and discomfort right now. This practice is designed to bring structural balance back into the body and gently stretch key muscle groups and thereby reduce pain and help you heal. The second practice is designed to build strength and flexibility and is more of a maintenance practice. This practice is recommended once pain has regularly subsided using the first practice — usually after 2 – 4 weeks. The second practice may also be used by anyone without active back problems who would like to prevent them in the future.

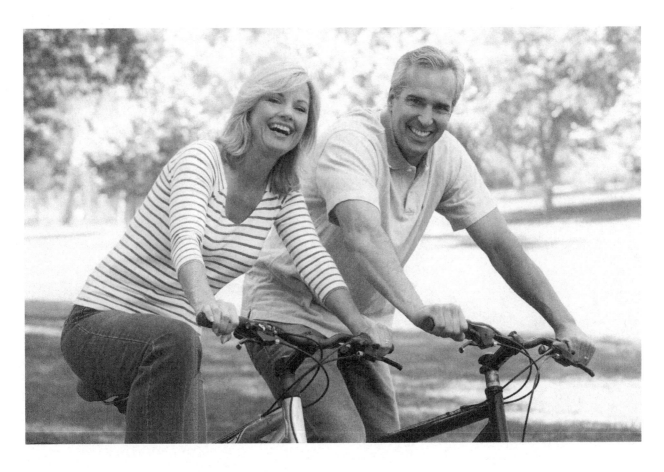

The bottom line is that the information in this book is going to help you get back into the activities and lifestyle you enjoy, without drugs, without costly treatments, in the comfort of your home, and you'll be more in control of your own health as well.

While it might be tempting to skip to the yoga section of the book, it is highly recommend that you read through the first few chapters as it will provide you with a lot of insight about back problems and make the yoga practice more meaningful.

Yoga therapy can help relieve

your pain while at the same time improve

your flexibility and strength, and get you back

into the activities you enjoy.

Chapter One

Causes of Lower Back Problems

In this chapter, we'll take a look at why so many people develop back problems. As you will discover, there are many reasons why back problems can occur, some of which are out of our control and some of which we actually have a lot of control over, such as lifestyle factors. In the next chapter, we will give you a brief overview of anatomy so you can get a clear picture of what is happening on the inside when you have back problems.

Accidents

One of the major causes of back problems is accidents. Take a moment to think about the ways accidents might happen:

- Slipping and falling down
- Tripping over the dog
- Missing a step on the stairs and falling down
- Climbing down from a ladder and missing the last rung
- Having a minor car accident…that little bump in a parking lot

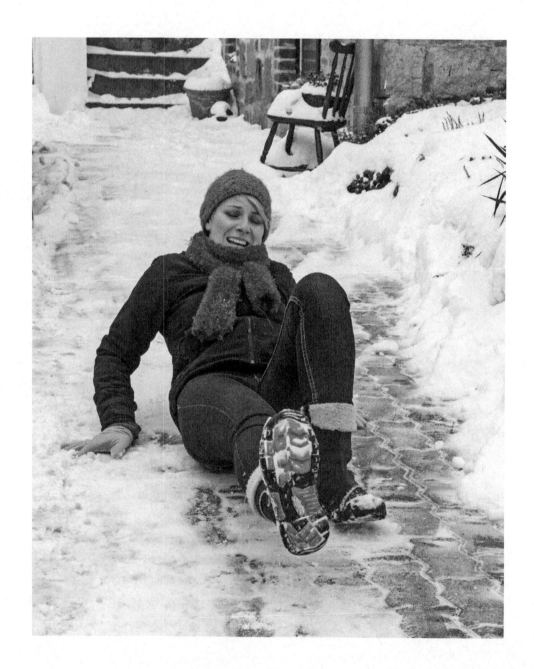

- Having a major car accident
- Sports injury
- Bumping into a door or a wall
- Stepping off a curb the wrong way
- Lifting a heavy package the wrong way

These are just a few of the more common accidents we hear about, but the way people have accidents is almost as diverse as people themselves.

The reason why accidents often lead to low back problems is that forces of the accident push the normal healthy functioning of your muscle-skeleton system out of balance. This imbalance may show up right away as excruciating pain, or it may not show up for weeks or months down the road.

Have you ever noticed a person walking with his or her leg in a cast? The added height of the cast will raise the hip on the side of the injury. Let's say you injured the right leg. The raised right hip will cause the spine to list to the left side away from vertical. You won't walk around bending to the left for very long because the muscle of the lower back will begin pulling your upper body back to the right, so that your eyes will be level. However your spine will now be twisted back to the right.

The muscle and ligaments of your spine will conform to the new position which will, in actuality, further cause strain and sprain. This will become your new "normal." When you get the cast off after a few weeks, your leg length will be level, however your spine will now be curved to the right. The ligaments and muscle will now have to adapt to the new position. Many times this can cause new or additional ligament and muscle pain. Proper rehabilitation of this area is essential and can be accomplished by a regular practice of yoga which will help provide a balance to the musculature.

Many people have an underlying problem that goes unnoticed for a long time until an accident does occur, exacerbating the condition and thus making itself known usually through pain or discomfort of some sort.

Lifestyle

Lifestyle choices also directly affect the health and functioning of the lower back. This is both bad news and good news. The bad news is that many of us are unwittingly doing things that contribute to or cause low back problems. The good news is that these lifestyle issues can all be addressed — with just a little effort.

Here are some common lifestyle issues that affect the health of the lower back:

- Sleeping
- Sitting
- Your choice of shoes
- Existing/Chronic injuries
- Pregnancy
- Lack of activity or exercise
- Carrying too much weight
- Wearing your wallet in your back pocket

Let's look at how these lifestyle factors affect your lower back:

SLEEPING ON YOUR STOMACH: Sleeping on your stomach will cause you to rotate your hip in such a way that you can actually strain your lower back, and it can lead to hip and knee pain. If you are sleeping on your stomach, we strongly advise either sleeping on your back or on your side with a pillow between your knees. This may feel weird at first, but give it a few nights and you will find it becomes familiar, and your back pain might just go away!

SITTING: What is your posture like when you watch television or sit at a computer? Do you sit upright with your torso over your hips and your feet flat on the floor, or do you slide down into your chair or sofa and put your feet up on the table? These positions put a lot of strain on the lower back.

Another position that many people slip into when at the computer is rounding their upper body forward and craning their neck forward. Sitting in this position for many hours every day puts a

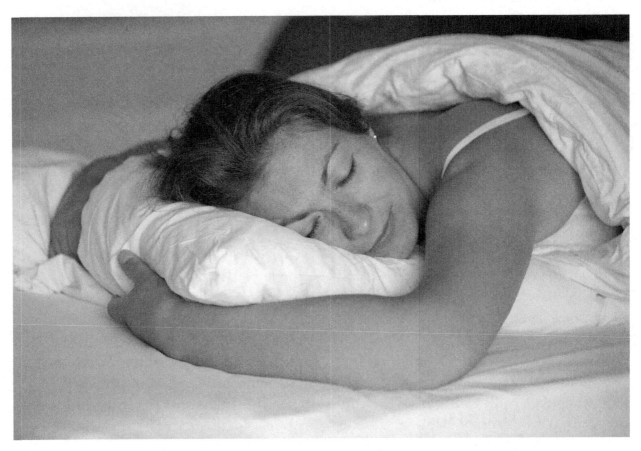

Sleeping on your stomach is the worst position for your back.

lot of strain on the lower back. Even with proper position, sitting for long periods of time can cause a lot of compression in your lower back. This is true for sitting in cars as well. You may be surprised to learn that most car seats are poorly designed to support your lower back.

If your job or lifestyle involves long periods of sitting, we highly recommend that you take a break every hour, go for a short walk, or do some gentle stretching.

NOTE: In the back of this book you will find a link for two **FREE** downloads: *Exercises You Can Do at Your Desk* and *Tips For Reducing Back And Repetitive Motion Injuries At Work*; especially good those who spend long hours on the computer!

SHOES: The kind and style of shoes you wear can greatly affect your back. Flats such as a ballet slipper style shoe for women (a minimal heel) or a boat/deck shoe for men often do not have a built-in arch to support your foot. Walking in this type of shoe will cause your foot to pronate while walking.

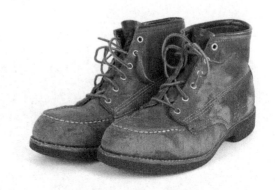

This gait alteration will cause your hip to rotate excessively which causes your back to compensate and twist.

Shoes with heels higher than one inch will cause the pelvis/hips to rotate forward causing the lumbosacral joint to "jam together." This jamming together of the facet joints causes tissue injury resulting in swelling, muscle spasm and tenderness in the low back. A person will usually have to sit down or perform low stretches to relieve the pain. As the body continues to experience this kind of recurring injury, early onset arthritis or more serious back issues can occur.

Wearing and walking in shoes with small pointed heels can also impede your normal gait because it produces a wobbly gait which interrupts the normal heel-toe movement that we all should have.

Wearing a shoe or shoes with excessively worn heels is another factor which produces low back pain. The wedging or wearing of the heel can alter your gait by causing an excessive roll in the normal heel toe portion of the gait. This will cause the affected hip to drop to the side, possibly jamming the sacroiliac joint and/or the lumbosacral joint.

EXISTING/CHRONIC INJURIES: Existing or prior hip, knee, foot, or ankle injuries can also contribute to low back pain. Injuries of these types can result in an abnormal gait which causes the hips to turn and the spine will compensate resulting in injury. A surgery that has become more and more common is hip replacement. Before the hip surgery the pelvis is usually out of alignment and the body has created a new normal position; the muscles and ligaments have adjusted to accommodate the altered structure.. After surgery, the pelvis is returned to a level position. Now, the lower back has to adjust to another new normal position. Related muscles and ligaments that were compensating for the chronic weak/injured hip now have to readjust and learn a new posture. A similar process takes place after any type of foot, ankle, or knee surgery.

Prior injuries to the lower back, resolved with or without surgery or proper rehabilitation, are another factor in recurring low back pain. Muscle and ligament tissue should be actively engaged for at least 120 days to allow proper rehabilitation. Many people think that once the pain is gone that everything is alright. In reality the healing process is only partially complete, and you are very vulnerable to re-injury during this phase of recovery. Sadly, we see all too many cases like this.

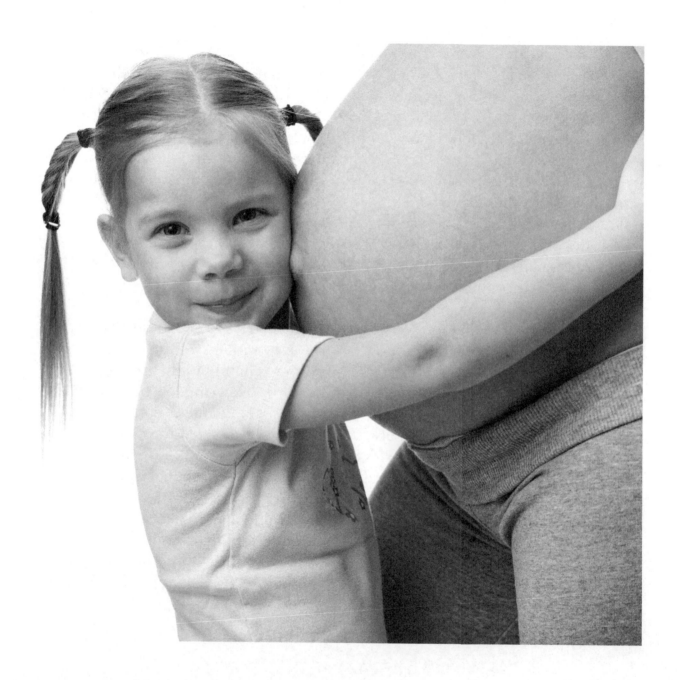

PREGNANCY: During pregnancy most women add an extra 10, 20, 30 or more pounds which adds a lot of stress to the musculoskeletal system. As the abdomen extends forward and down, the low back/lumbar spine curves forward. This extension causes the lumbar and lumbosacral facets to jam together. As the baby continues to grow and begins to turn, pressure can also be put into the pelvis area causing the sacroiliac joint to spread and the hips compensate. Many times the sacrum will also rotate and the hips twist causing the sciatic nerve to become involve.

Once a woman gives birth, a whole new series of factors can influence the low back. The baby is now carried around in the arms of mom or dad. New upper body weight distribution (carrying the baby) causes the lower back to compensate and work harder as mom or dad gets used to lifting the baby in or out of the car seat, crib, or carrying the baby in the back pack. Every day household activities such as resting the little one on the mother's hip while cooking, vacuuming, doing the dishes, talking on the phone, all put tremendous strain on the lower back.

For the mother, sacroiliac joints on both side of the sacrum can be very "loose" at this time as well. As a woman's body begins to recover from pregnancy, the ligaments and muscle of the lower back/pelvis and abdomen begin to tighten and return to their pre-pregnancy state. If the bones are not in proper alignment with the ligaments and muscles, they may heal in an abnormal position. Early attention to the area with yoga can help bring this balance to the lower back.

LACK OF EXERCISE/ACTIVITY: Perhaps one the most effective way to keep your spine healthy and pain free is with regular movement which introduces flexibility and strengthening. It also helps to remove stress which helps the body regain balance. We were born to move! Lack of exercise has the opposite effect: the body becomes weaker, less flexible, and imbalances stay in the body — all of which sets you up for injury.

We are not suggesting that you need to engage in two hours of aerobics and body building every day to get the benefits of movement. On the contrary, some gentle yoga and walking will do the trick. Shoot for 20 – 30 minutes four to five times per week.

And a word to weekend warriors: be sure to take time to warm up before your activities and cool down after. Doing a few of the yoga postures in this book before or after your activity is a great way to prevent injuries.

MAINTAINING A HEALTHY WEIGHT: Study after study shows that people who are overweight are at greater risk for back pain, joint pain, and muscle strain than those who are not. There are a number of reasons for this. First, extra weight can pull on the spine and surrounding structures causing them to tilt or become stressed unevenly. This adds strain to the joints, muscles, and ligaments of the spine and surrounding areas. Over time, the back can lose its support and functioning, and an unnatural curvature of the spine may develop.

Secondly, for every extra pound of weight on the body there is a corresponding increase in load on the joints of the body. Too much load results in wear and tear of these joints, leading to serious complications such as the wearing away of cartilage, bulging discs, arthritis, and increased pain. Simply put: extra weight puts extra stress on your body.

Thirdly, most people who are overweight or obese are not engaging in enough exercise or enough activity to keep their weight down. As far as back care goes, this is tragic because, as mentioned above, the right kind of physical activity is both the prevention and cure for most back issues.

Additionally, people who are overweight are more likely to feel pain in their body due to systemic inflammation associated with extra weight and a diet high in inflammatory foods. So not exercising and being overweight in and of itself can have a spiraling down effect on a person's overall health and, as well, their spine.

While it is not the focus of this book to recommend a specific nutrition plan, we do advise that a sound nutrition or diet plan contain the following key components:

1. Lose weight slowly — studies show that people who drop pounds slowly over time tend to keep it off longer. 1 to 2 lbs. per week is a good goal.

2. Look for diets that feature whole foods rather than processed or packaged food. Look for fresh vegetables, fruits, whole grains, legumes, and lowfat proteins such as chicken, turkey, fish, etc. These foods will give you the nutrition your body needs to function properly and help reduce any inflammation or pain in your body. Avoid products with white flour, sugar, high fructose corn syrup, and hydrogenated oils. These products lack any nutritional value and cause inflammation.

3. Avoid extreme diets. Diets such as ultra-low carb, lowfat, ultra-low calorie or high protein eliminate key food groups, and you end up craving them — then most likely binging! So look for a diet that is balanced with approximately 25–30% of calories coming from fat and 25–30% coming from protein.

WALLET IN BACK POCKET: This one is mostly for the guys because we are the ones most often doing this! Yes, it is convenient, but when you sit on your wallet you cause one hip to be higher than the other which results in stress on your hip joints, sacroiliac joints, and your spine. This can either cause an injury or make an existing one worse. So, take the wallet out of your back pocket!

Genetic / Congenital

While scientists cannot agree as to whether lower back problems can be passed on genetically, they can agree that it can be common for members of a family to have similar back problems. For example, suppose my grandfather was a farmer, my dad was a farmer, and I am a farmer. We are all right-handed and drove the same tractor; we would, in all likelihood, develop the same low back problems.

This can be due primarily to biological and mechanical factors (musculoskeletal) as well as lifestyle factors as indicated above that family members may share.

We may also come into the world with certain physical conditions that will lead to lower back problems such as scoliosis, having one leg longer than the other, etc.

Disease Factors

The human body can be subject to neuro-muscular diseases which can affect the back. For example: Polio, a neurologic disease may result in muscle wasting on one or both sides of the body. As the patient recovers from this disease the muscular wasting may affect one side more than the other creating an imbalance. The body will then attempt to compensate for the imbalance and excessive strain will be placed on the joints of the low back. The person will "get by" with what may be an altered gait and general weakness in the lower back. As they age, the body in its wisdom, may try to compensate for this weakness by depositing bone (creating bone spurs/osteophytes) in the lumbar spine to gain stability. This can be viewed as another disease process rather than the body's attempt to help.

Multiple sclerosis (MS) is a disease that affects the brain and spinal cord resulting in loss of muscle control as well as other symptoms. The loss of communication from the brain to the affected musculature can cause an imbalance to occur affecting one side of the low back more than the other. Through the a regular yoga practice, the body brain communication can be reinforced and perhaps strengthened along with the affected musculature.

Fibromyalgia, a diagnosis relatively new in the health care community is an apparent neuromuscular problem affecting the entire body. When the lower back is involved, a generalized aching lack of strength and endurance are common symptoms. With a general malaise and constant aching throughout the body occurring, musculature imbalance can occur contributing the recurring low back problem. A regular and gentle practice of yoga can help reduce symptoms and move the patient to recovery Existing arthritic changes already in the body, the result of any long standing musculature imbalance, may also contribute to the acute low back problem.

Combination of Factors

Obviously, any of the issues just mentioned can be the direct or indirect cause of lower back problems. Often, however, multiple factors exist at the same time making the situation worse. For example, let's say that John has arthritis in his lower back, spends a lot of time driving in his car, and then comes home at night to sit in front of the sofa watching television for a couple hours. Add to this that he is a stomach sleeper and you can begin to see how his lifestyle can be negatively impacting an underlying problem.

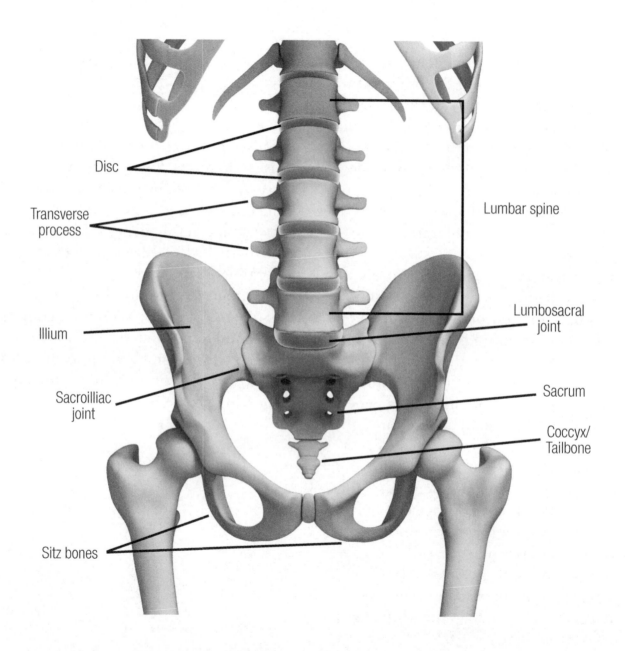

Disc

Transverse
process

Lumbar spine

Illium

Lumbosacral
joint

Sacroilliac
joint

Sacrum

Coccyx/
Tailbone

Sitz bones

Chapter Two

Anatomy of the Low Back

In this chapter, we offer you a brief review of anatomy. We do this so you can begin to understand the structure of your body and how it is supposed to work. Then, in the next chapter, you will see what happens inside your body when you have a lower back problem.

For the purposes of our discussion, the low back consist of the 5 lumbar vertebra, the sacrum, the coccyx (tailbone) and the right and left ilium (right and left hip). Also included are the vertebral disc, the lumbosacral joint, the sacroiliac joint, the facet joints, and the ligaments and muscles of the low back.

The purpose of the lumbar spine is to provide mobility for the rest of the back. It also furnishes support for the upper portion of the body and transmits weight to the pelvis and lower extremities. The lumbar spine has a relatively wide range of motion.

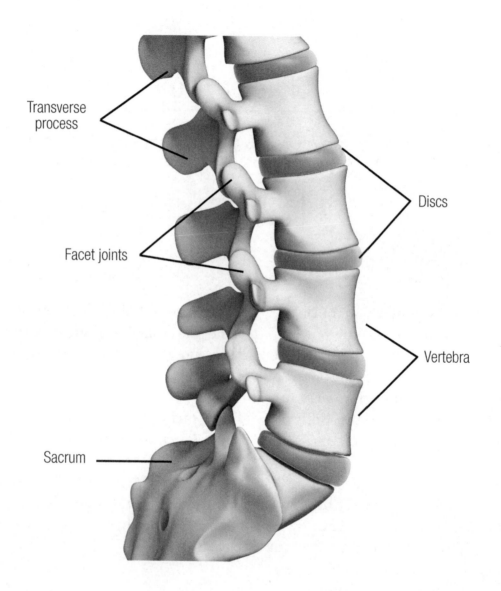

Transverse
process

Facet joints

Sacrum

Discs

Vertebra

You'll notice that the 5 vertebras stacked one on top of the other. The vertebra consists of the body, the spinous process, 2 transverse processes, and 2 facet joints. Each vertebrae is separated by the disc.

The facet joints at the back of the body serve to guide the vertebra as they bend forward, backward, sideways, and twist.

The 5 stacked vertebra rest on the flat or top end of the sacrum. The joint created by the vertebra and sacrum is called the lumbosacral joint. (Just a side note: this joint is designed to support the entire upper body.)

Looking further at the lower back, we can see that the sacrum is attached to the right and left hip. The joint created by this union is called the sacroiliac joint, often referred to as the SI joint.

The joints we mentioned before …the facet joints …the lumbosacral joint and the sacroiliac joint are all held together by various ligaments. Ligaments are fibrous connective tissue that connects bone to bone.

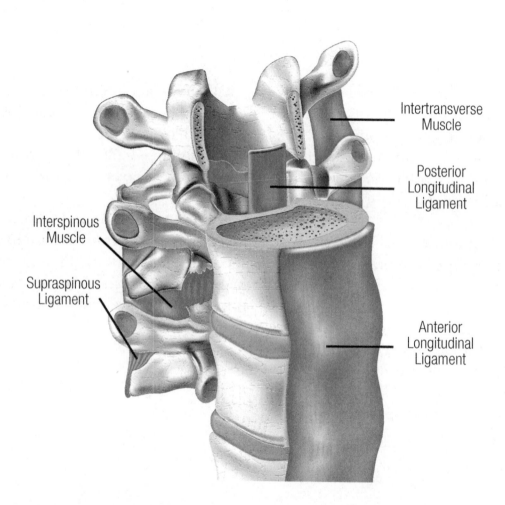

Intertransverse
Muscle

Posterior
Longitudinal
Ligament

Interspinous
Muscle

Supraspinous
Ligament

Anterior
Longitudinal
Ligament

Small tiny ligaments connect all of the
lumbar vertebrae together at the facet
joints. Larger broad base ligaments
connect the hips and sacrum together,
giving the lower back a very stable base
to support the body.

Two more very important ligaments
that we rarely hear about until we
have a significant problem are the
anterior (front) and the posterior
(back) longitudinal ligaments. These
ligaments connect the vertebra
together at the front of the body and
the back of the body. These ligaments
extend from the top of the neck to
the tailbone and serve to stabilize the
entire spinal column.

The spinal disc/intervertebral disc serve
as natural shock absorbers cushioning
and separating the vertebra from each
other. The disc is composed of two parts:
the nucleus and the annulus fibrosus
which forms a woven jelly-like filled
cushion attached to the bottom of one
vertebra and the top of the next vertebra.
The annulus also forms the tough outer

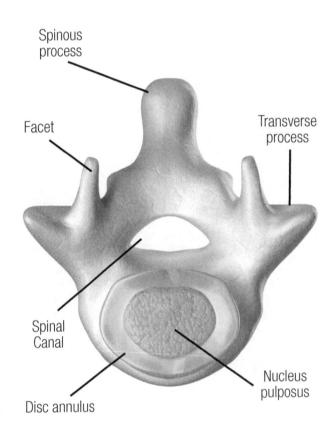

Spinous
process

Facet

Transverse
process

Spinal
Canal

Disc annulus

Nucleus
pulposus

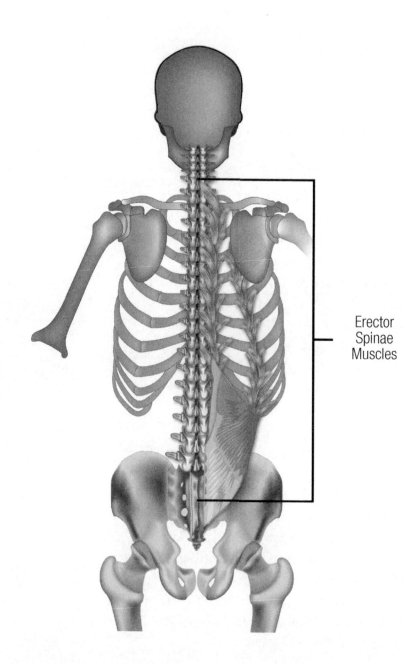

Erector
Spinae
Muscles

wall of the disc itself. The nucleus sits in the center of the disc and serves much like a ball bearing around which the vertebral body can move. The helps provide for an overall flexible spine.

Lastly, there are the major muscle groups most often involved in lower back pain and injuries:

The lower back includes the *erector spinae group* attaches on both sides of the back at the sacrum and then at the specific spinous and transverse processes throughout the spinal column. This muscle group extends into the upper back and neck.

This group of muscles allows flexion and extension (forward and backward motion) of the spinal column. The *erector spinae group* also functions to draw the head and ribs down as well as permit lateral flexion (movement to the other side) of the trunk.

Psoas
Muscle

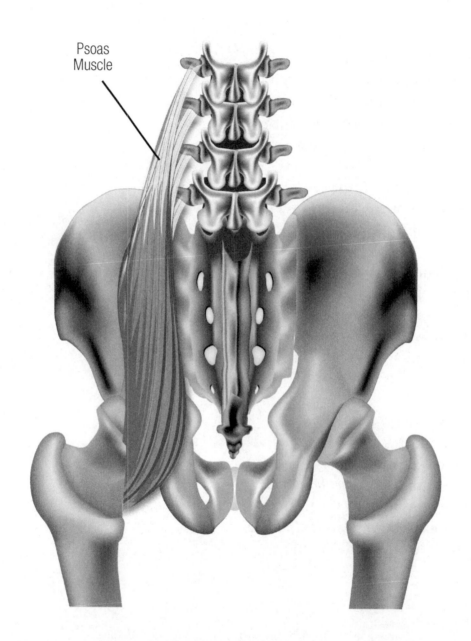

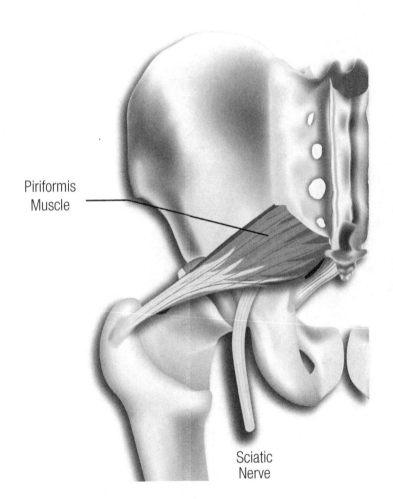

Piriformis
Muscle

Sciatic
Nerve

The psoas muscle attaches on the front of the lumbar spine and into the inner leg. This muscle provided stability to the lower trunk allowing hip rotation and flexion.

The piriformis muscle attaches to the sacrum and then into the leg. This muscle helps provide hip rotation and is critical to the body weight shifting from the right side to the left side while walking.

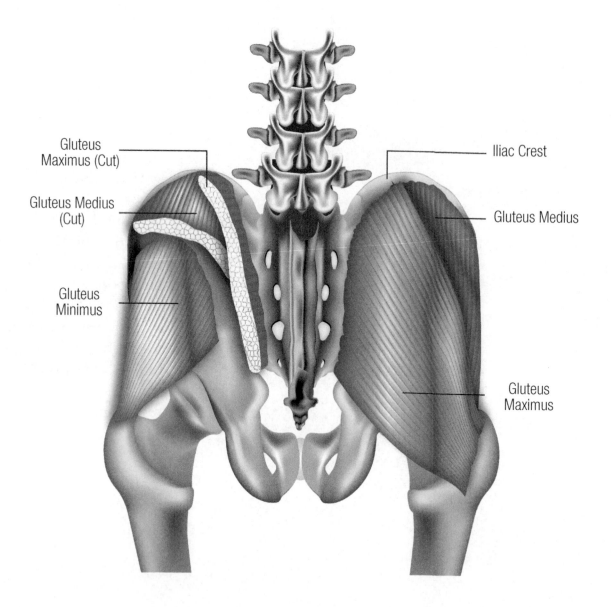

Gluteus
Maximus (Cut)

Gluteus Medius
(Cut)

Gluteus
Minimus

Iliac Crest

Gluteus Medius

Gluteus
Maximus

The *buttock or gluteus muscle* group,
composed of the gluteus maximus,
medius and minimus, attach at the hip,
sacrum, and into the legs. These muscles
serve to support the entire lower body,
providing stability to the trunk for
standing, walking, and sitting.

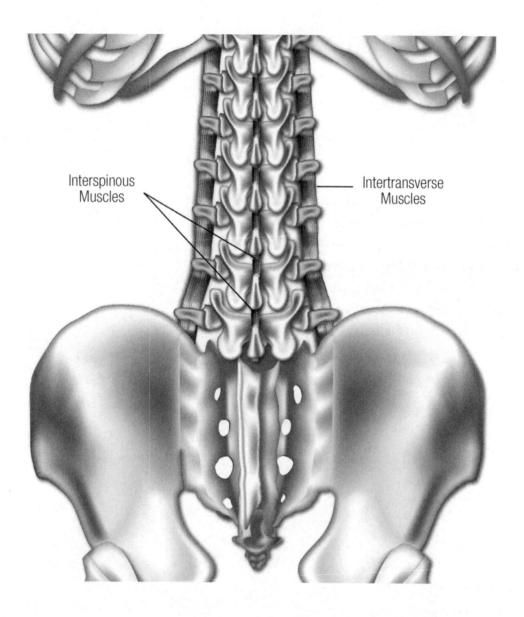

Interspinous
Muscles

Intertransverse
Muscles

Finally, there are the very tiny but
extremely important interspinous and
intertransverse muscles. These tiny
muscles extend from one process to
another, sometimes connecting spinous
to spinous, transverse to transverse, or
spinous to transverse. Sometimes they
will even skip the vertebra directly below
to attach to a lower area to facilitate
spinal movement. This small muscle
provides movement to each of the
vertebra and, therefore, provides the
intricate movement of the entire spinal
column.

Now that you have an understanding of
what's on the inside, let's take a look at
what goes wrong and how that creates
the lower back pain.

The purpose of the lumbar spine is to provide mobility for the rest of the back. It also furnishes support for the upper portion of the body and transmits weight to the pelvis and lower extremities.

Chapter Three

Common Lower Back Problems— What's going on inside?

In this chapter, we will take a look at common lower back problems and discuss what is actually happening inside when these problems occur.

Sprain/Strain

The most common injury to the lower back is the sprain/strain of the lower back ligaments and/or musculature. We many times refer to this as a "muscle pull." This type on injury typically occurs when we fall down, lift something awkwardly, or sit or sleep with poor posture.

When a sprain occurs, the ligaments, the fibrous connective tissue holding the bones/joints together, will stretch beyond their normal capacity. If severe enough, the fibers can even tear apart.

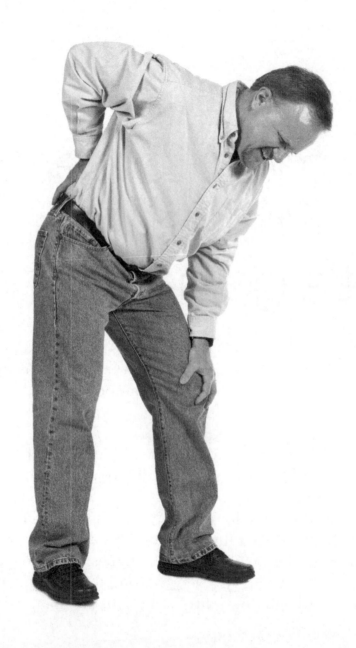

The body reacts by swelling in the area of injury, pain receptors fire off, and muscles will spasm.

A strain occurs in muscle and can be caused by the same type of action that causes the ligament to sprain. Small micro-tears occur in the muscle fibers causing pain, swelling, tenderness, and weakness to develop at the sight of injury.

Repetitive strain/sprain injuries to the same area will result in a weakening of the ligament and muscles. Chronic sprains and degenerative changes such as osteoarthritis of the spine are very commonly the result of repetitive injuries.

Facet Joint Injuries

As described in the last chapter, these are the tiny joints on the back of the vertebral body. When you bend too far forward, twist too far to the right or left, or simply hold the facet in the wrong position for too long, the ligaments can sprain or tear. For example, by sleeping on your stomach you can actually sprain the ligaments that connect the facet joints together on one side of the spine and jam together the facet joints on the other side. When this happens, swelling occurs, tissue tears, and pain results.

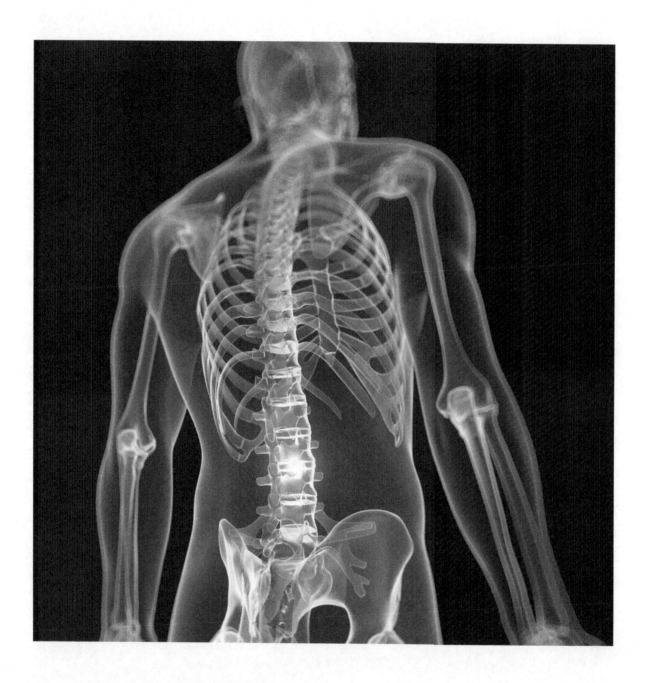

Discs Injuries

The more serious injuries to the lower back involve the spinal disc. If you remember from our earlier discussion, the discs sit between the vertebral bodies connecting the vertebra together.

The trauma we receive from falls, missed steps, sports injuries, auto accidents, and even poor postural position will all contribute to the gradual weakening and tearing of the disc fibers (annulus pulposus). As the disc weakens, the nucleus can shift position.

When this happens, the structure of the spinal column is changed, causing the rest of the lower back to compensate. The spine, in the area of the injured disc, will twist or turn in an attempt by your body to achieve balance. Muscles above and below the injury will spasm, creating more stress on the ligaments and surrounding bone structures.

As the disc continues to tear and weaken, the jelly-like cushion inside the disc can move to the back, the side, or the front of the disc. When the disc material begins to reach the outer margins of the disc, it becomes painful and is referred to as a bulging disc. If the injured disc continues to be traumatized, it can herniate or rupture into the spinal canal, creating even more serious complications involving the spinal cord and nerves.

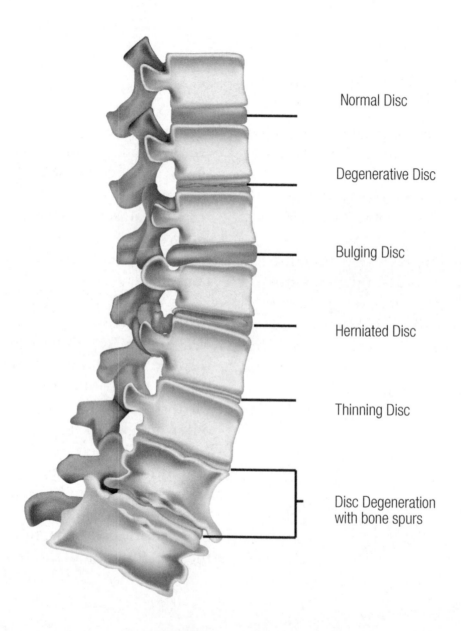

Normal Disc

Degenerative Disc

Bulging Disc

Herniated Disc

Thinning Disc

Disc Degeneration
with bone spurs

Common disk problems

A DEGENERATED DISC is a natural and normal part of the aging process and is very common. The disc loses its natural height and stature through dehydration, lack of nourishment, and lack of motion. The degenerative disc then causes chronic back pain by compressing the nerve roots and giving the spinal cord and nerves less room to function normally. Adjacent tissue can also become involved resulting in additional pain and inflammation.

A BULGING DISC IS A DISC that has begun to lose it structural integrity. That may have occurred due to acute trauma or repetitive micro trauma. The annular fibers of the internal disc may be torn allowing the nucleus to begin migratingto the outer boarders of the disc pressing against the outer annular fibers. This can cause nerve pressure on the spinal cord and adjacent nerves, resulting in pain and nerve impairment.

A HERNIATED DISC is a disc that has suffered a disruption of the tough outer fibers of the annulus fibrosis. The material of the nucleus pulposes then breaks through the outer wall of the disc and may be pressing into the spinal canal or the intervertebral foramina of the spine. This is usually very painful, producing possible neurological impingement.

DISC DEGENERATION with spur formation is a natural occurring process that the body performs in an attempt to restore stability to the spine. Though a naturally occurring process, this condition can be the result of repetitive trauma, micro trauma, lack of proper spinal motion, muscle imbalance, or poor nutrition.

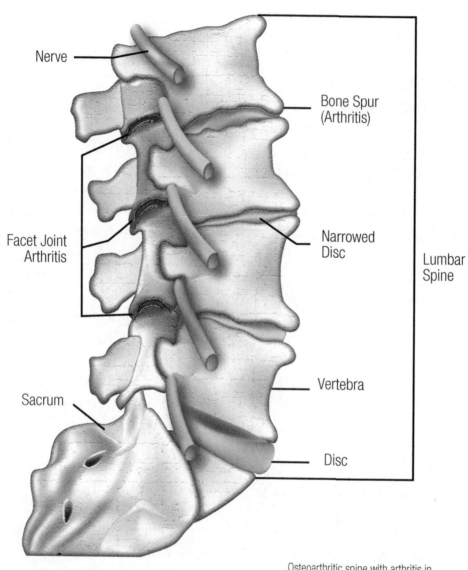

Nerve

Bone Spur
(Arthritis)

Facet Joint
Arthritis

Narrowed
Disc

Lumbar
Spine

Sacrum

Vertebra

Disc

Osteoarthritic spine with arthritis in
vertebrae & facet joints

Spinal Arthritis

Spinal arthritis, commonly referred to as osteoarthritis, is actually a very common and accepted part of aging. Referring to this condition as spondylosis and degenerative joint disease is also quite common.

The arthritis of the lumbar spine is usually the result of repetitive micro-traumas to the ligaments, discs, and facet joints of the lumbar vertebra (lower back). As the ligaments weaken due to repetitive trauma, disc degeneration occurs. This brings the vertebra closer together. As the vertebra come closer together, the facet joints begin to stress/rub together. This weakened state causes the body to replace damaged soft tissue with bone. The vertebra begin to soften at the borders as bone is moved into the damaged tissue. This is done as an attempt by the body to strengthen and limit further damage to the joint.

We call these calcifications bone spurs or osteophytes. The spurs can develop at most any place that ligaments are damaged, not only in the major joints but also in the small tiny facet joints. When vertebral spurs are left untreated they will eventually fuse together, severely limiting the movement of the spine.

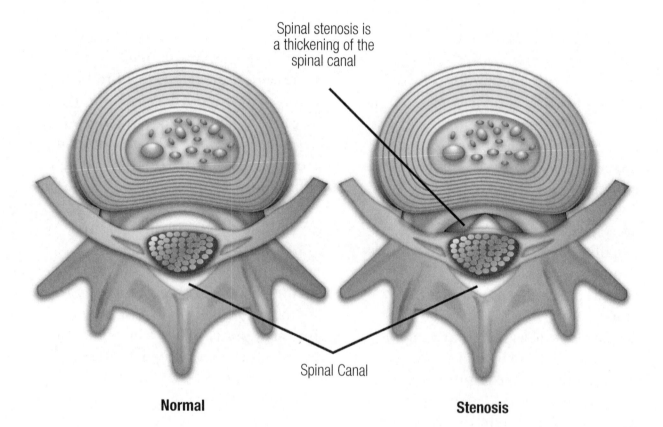

Spinal stenosis is a thickening of the spinal canal

Spinal Canal

Normal

Stenosis

Spinal Stenosis: What is it?

Many times we see patients and clients who have recently been informed that they have spinal stenosis. This usually happens following a recent episode of lower back pain and visit to their physician who has recommended a MRI study.

Spinal stenosis is the narrowing of the spinal canal usually caused by the thickening of the posterior longitudinal ligament, disc bulging, and possible spur formation. The development of stenosis will many times result in back pain, loss of movement, and loss of motor function.

Sciatica

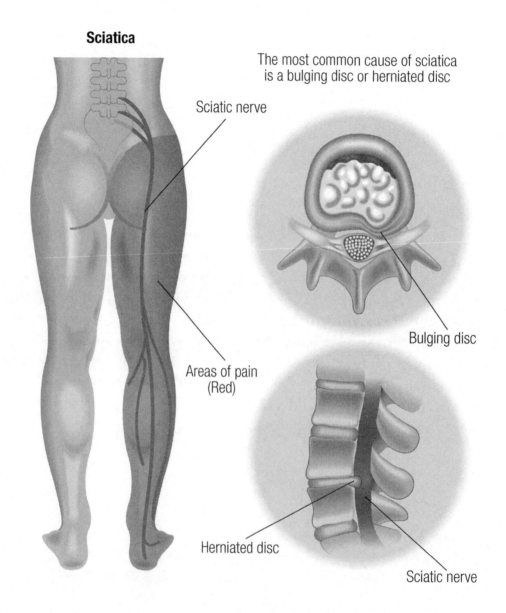

The most common cause of sciatica is a bulging disc or herniated disc

Sciatic nerve

Areas of pain (Red)

Bulging disc

Herniated disc

Sciatic nerve

Sciatica

The term sciatica refers to the radiating pain brought on the by the inflammation of the largest and longest nerve in the body.

The sciatic nerve is composed of the nerve roots from the L4-5, L5-S1, S1-S2, S2-S3 vertabra. Bilateral branches run down both legs and break up to form the peripheral nerve system which provides the sensory and motor functions of the buttocks/legs and feet.

The sciatic nerve is about the diameter/width of your little finger. It lays across the sacroiliac joint, passes under the piriformis muscle, exits the pelvis through the sciatic notch of the ilium (hip), and runs down the back of the leg.

True sciatica is caused by the compression of one or more of the specific nerve roots mentioned above; therefore, injuries to the vertebra, discs, surrounding muscle, and sacroiliac joint can all contribute to the development of sciatic nerve pain.

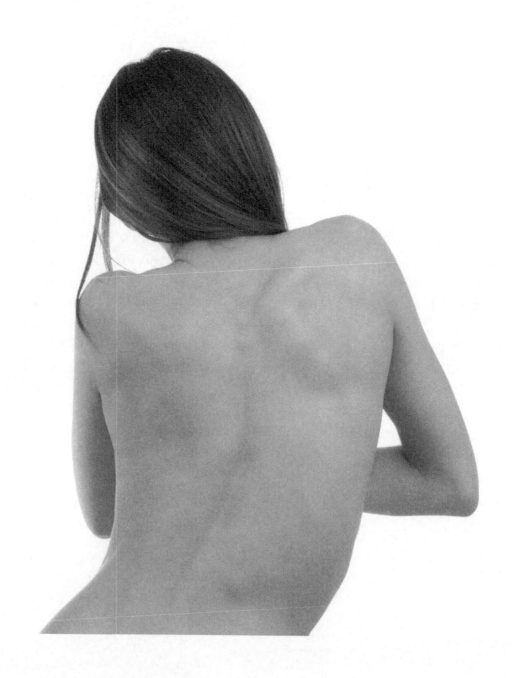

Scoliosis

Scoliosis, or curvature of the spine, is
a condition when the spinal column
can turn from the neck to the sacrum.
Its origin can be congenital, that is to
say genetic; you are simply born with a
vertebra anomaly, and as you grow your
spine twists and curves as it attempts to
achieve balance. This type of scoliosis
is not very common; however, the most
commonly seen form of scoliosis is the
result of a spinal muscle imbalance
most often caused by a structural
change. Remember those simple
falls, and the poor sleeping or sitting
postures? These can all be linked to the
development of scoliosis.

Hyperlordosis

Lordosis refers to the inward curvature of a portion of the lumbar and cervical vertebral column. While it is normal to have some lordosis, "hyperlordosis," sometimes called "swayback," refers to an excessive inward curving of the lumbar spine. Left untreated, hyperlordosis can lead to disc injury, facet jamming, spinal stenosis, and spinal cord pressure. Common causes of hyperlordosis are tight lower back muscles, weak hamstrings, or tight hip flexors (psoas).

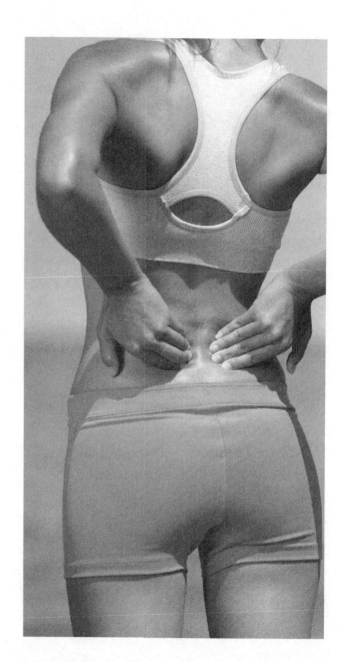

Chapter Four

Lifestyle Tips

In this chapter, we will offer lifestyle tips that you can implement to maintain and enhance the progress you are making with your back.

AVOID SLEEPING ON YOUR STOMACH: If you are a stomach sleeper, "don't!" Sleeping on your stomach is one of the worst positions you can put yourself into for your lower back. When you lay on your stomach, you first have to turn your head to the right or left, twisting your neck and upper back in such a way as to stress the disc, ligaments, facet joints, and muscles.

Can you imagine going to the movies sitting sideways and then attempting to watch the movie? Imagine what your neck would feel like after just a few minutes.

This is what happens in the low back when you sleep on your stomach. First, the weight of the spine, approximately 15 lbs., is resting on your internal organs: stomach, large, and small intestine.

Secondly, you will have to draw your right or left leg up, twisting your hips/pelvis and rotating your hip/leg. This position adds stress to the hip socket, knee, and the sacroiliac joint. As the sacroiliac joint continues to be stressed, the lumbosacral joint connecting the sacrum becomes involved. This in turn will create facet and disc stress and damage, which are an early cause of low back pain.

Well, then, how should you sleep? Sleeping on your side or back is one of the most beneficial lifestyle changes you can make. However, this can also be challenging because so many of you may have slept on your stomach since childhood and developed a strong habit. To make the change to sleeping on your side easier, simply lay on your side in a fetal position, place a small pillow or folded towel between your knees, hug a pillow to your chest, and you will be able to get a good night's sleep without compromising your lower back.

LIMIT YOUR SITTING AT A COMPUTER OR IN DRIVING TO 40 MINUTES: Stand up if working at a computer or stop and get out of the car and walk around for a few minutes.

Set a timer to remind you if necessary. If you are watching TV, stand up after every other set of the commercials.

FLEX YOUR KNEES WHEN STANDING AT THE SINK WHILE WASHING OR BRUSHING YOUR TEETH: When standing at the kitchen sink washing dishes, open the cabinet door and place a foot on the inside shelf, taking the pressure off your low back.

AVOID CROSSING YOUR LEGS: This stops your hips and sacroiliac joint from straining and your lower back from twisting.

USE YOUR LEGS WHEN GETTING OUT OF A CHAIR: Move forward to the front of the chair and place a foot underneath the chair. Keeping your back straight use your legs to gently raise to an upright position.

WEAR SUPPORTIVE AND PROPER FITTING SHOES: Check the heels of your shoes for unusual wear patterns. Fix them or replace them. Use shoe orthotics or inserts to support your arches. Avoid wearing high heels as much as possible as they can negatively affect your posture.

APPLY ICE OR MOIST HEAT TO YOUR LOWER BACK FOLLOWING ANY STRENUOUS ACTIVITY: Follow the simple formula presented in the chapter on low back first aid.

TAKE SOME DEEP BREATHS: Breathe in through your nose out letting your belly expand as you inhale. As you exhale and move your bellybutton towards your spine. Do this many times throughout the day. This will help your posture, keep you relaxed, and help ease pain.

STAY HYDRATED — DRINK PLENTY OF WATER THROUGHOUT THE DAY. 6 TO 8 GLASSES (12OZ.): This helps keep your tissues plump and functioning well.

DEVELOP A REGULAR WALKING ROUTINE: Next to a regular practice of yoga, walking is one of the easiest and most cost effective lifestyle habits you can use to regain your health and vitality.

PRACTICE THE YOGA POSTURES RECOMMENDED IN THIS BOOK REGULARLY: It is the regular practice over time that produces the most benefits.

Yoga is a practice for the entire mind and body

which means that not only is it helpful for your low back,

but it can also help you are sleep better,

improve your mood, and you'll enjoy

an enhanced sense of overall well-being.

Chapter Five

Yoga for Relieving Low Back Pain

In this book, we are presenting two levels of yoga practice. The first level is for people who are experiencing acute symptoms — that is, you are in pain right now. The second level is added to the first sequence to help strengthen and build more flexibility in your lower back.

If you are in the acute phase, we recommend that you do the first sequence daily for 2–4 weeks or longer before adding the strengthening and flexibility phase.

You'll know you are ready for the second phase because you are experiencing little or no discomfort in your lower back on a day to day basis.

The second level is also ideal if your lower back symptoms tend to come and go over time, or if you just want to proactively build strength and flexibility in your back.

In any case, you should **always** begin your practice with the first sequence and move to the second only when you are ready.

If you are in pain, we recommend that you practice the first section once or twice daily.

As you begin your practice — always remember to never do anything that causes you pain. It is ok to feel some mild stretching sensations, which is good, but never force your body to do something that doesn't feel right.

For your practice, ideally you'll want to be on a yoga mat or at least on a carpeted surface. If you are working on a hard wood floor and don't have a mat, then a large thick towel or small blanket will work for now.

It is also helpful to have a few yoga props nearby: a yoga strap, or if you don't have a strap, a bath towel or old tie can work equally well. Having a thick blanket and yoga block will also come in handy.

As you begin your practice — always remember

to never do anything that causes you pain.

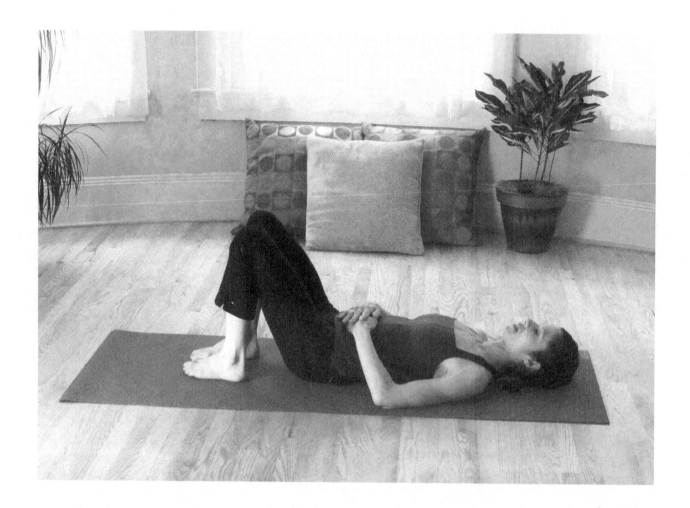

Breathing

GOING INTO THE POSTURE:
We are going to begin with some belly breathing.

Start by laying on your back, bending your knees and placing your feet on the floor. Have your thighs in line with your hips. Now place your hands on your belly.

As you inhale, breath in through your nose and let your belly expand up into your hands. As you exhale through your nose, release your belly button towards your spine. Inhale through your nose and let your belly expand, and then exhale through your nose and release. Inhale, big belly, exhale releasing your belly button towards your spine. If your nose is clogged, it is ok to breathe slowly through your mouth.

Now slow your breath a little more — making it smooth on the inhale and smooth on the exhale. Continue breathing in this fashion.

BENEFITS: Belly breathing gently moves the spine — introducing movement. Belly breathing also helps to relax tight muscles, reduces pain in your body, and brings oxygen into your system. Take a couple more breaths. Notice how your body and mind may have already begun to relax.

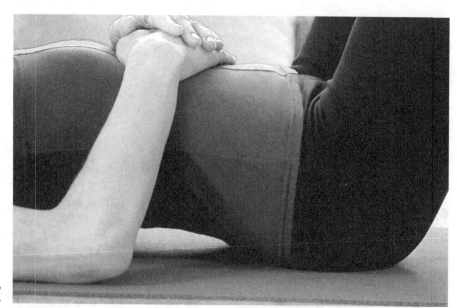

As you inhale, roll your hips forward, pressing your tailbone into the floor.

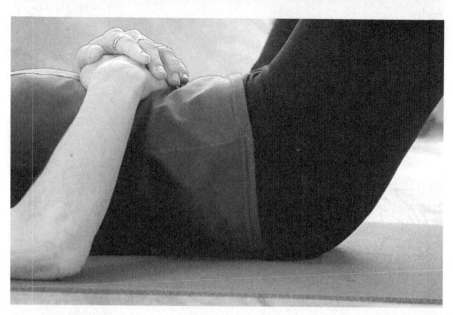

As you exhale, roll your hips back towards your torso, pressing the top of your sacrum into the floor.

Pelvic tilts

GOING INTO THE POSTURE:
Staying on your back with your feet on the floor, you are going to tilt the top of your pelvic area forward so that your tailbone presses into the floor; do this as you slowly inhale. As you exhale, rotate your hips back so that the top of your sacrum presses into the floor.

As you slowly inhale, rock your hips forward, pressing your tailbone towards the floor. As you slowly exhale, rotate your hips back, pressing the top of the sacrum towards the floor. Repeat this sequence several times — coordinating the movement with your breath.

BENEFITS: This exercise is very good for gently stretching and strengthening your lower back and for bringing flexibility to your spine and hips. It also helps to improve circulation to your hips, lower back, and pelvic area.

As you inhale, roll your hips forward, pressing your tailbone into the floor.

As you exhale, roll your hips back towards your torso, pressing the top of your sacrum into the floor.

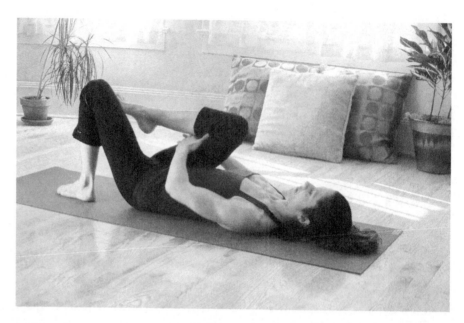

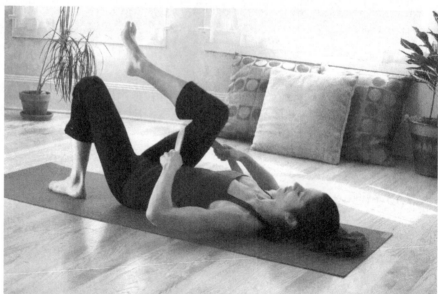

Reclining knee to chest
pose using a strap.

Reclining knee to chest

GOING INTO THE POSTURE:
Lay on the floor with feet flat on the floor and both knees bent, bring your right knee into your chest, interlace your fingers around the back of your right thigh and bring your right knee further towards your chest. If your hands don't easily reach the back of your thigh, then place a yoga strap or small towel behind your thigh and grab the sides of the strap or towel as shown.

Now, slowly extend your left leg onto the floor and stretch through your left heel. If you feel any discomfort in your lower back hips, keep the left knee bent instead of straightening it onto the floor.

Take 5 to 10 long slow breaths. Remember to breathe in through your nose — expanding your belly and breathe out through your nose, releasing your belly button towards your spine.

COMING OUT OF THE POSTURE: Now, release your right foot to the floor and bring your left knee into your chest, interlace your fingers behind your thigh, and draw your left thigh towards your chest.

Slowly extend the right leg onto the floor and extend through the right heel. If you feel any discomfort then bend your right knee, placing your right foot on the floor.

Take 5 to 10 long slow breaths — breathing in through your nose and out through your nose.

BENEFITS: This posture is particularly good for stretching your lower back, bringing flexibility to your hips, and is good for your digestion as well.

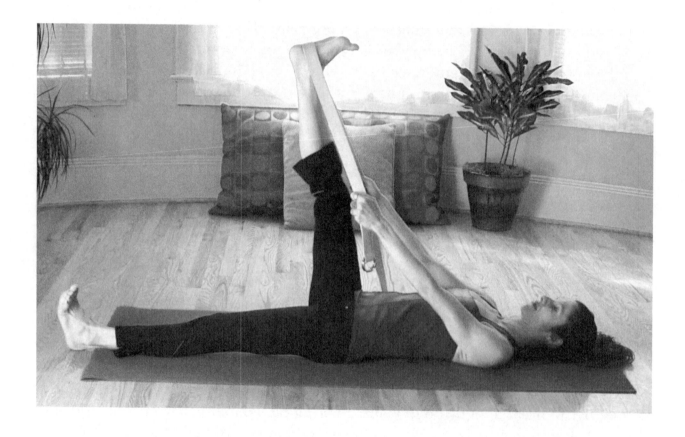

Reclining hamstring stretch

GOING INTO THE POSTURE:
For this posture, you will need your yoga strap or towel.

Lay on your back with your legs extended onto the floor. Have your strap or towel in your hands. Bring your feet together, bring your big toes together, and bring your heels together. Stretch through your heels, pressing your thigh bones down towards the floor.

Take in a deep breath. As you exhale, bring your right knee into your chest and place the belt or towel around your right heel, and then slowly extend your right leg up towards the ceiling, letting the strap slide through your hands.

Ideally, you want your right leg straight, but if your hamstrings are tight, you will find this hard to do. If you do have tight hamstrings, let the strap slide through your hands a little and let your right leg drop a little towards the floor until it straightens.

You should feel a mild stretching sensation in the back of the thigh and maybe the calf. Make sure you are not feeling the stretch in the back of the knee. If you do feel it here, you will need to drop the right leg further toward the floor.

Now, stretch through your left heel, drawing your toes towards your face, and press your left thighbone down towards the floor. Reach up through your right heel into the strap.

If you have any discomfort in your lower back or sacroiliac joint area while doing this exercise, try bending your left knee and placing your left foot on the floor. If you still have discomfort, then don't do this posture and go onto the next.

Relax your shoulders, relax your neck, and relax your facial muscles. Take 5 to 10 long slow deep breaths. Remember to breathe in through your nose and out through your nose, letting your belly expand as you inhale and release as you exhale.

COMING OUT OF THE POSTURE: On your last breath, slowly flex your knee. Release your belt and lower your right leg/foot to the floor. And now you will do the left side.

GOING INTO THE POSTURE: Extend both legs onto the floor. Bring your feet together, bringing your big toes together and your heels together. Stretch through your heels. Press your thigh bones down towards the floor.

Take in a deep breath. As you exhale, bring your left knee into your chest and place the belt or towel around your left heel, and then slowly extend your left leg up towards the ceiling, letting the strap slide through your hands.

Now, stretch through your right heel and press your right thigh down towards the floor. Reach up through your left heel into the strap.

Remember, if you have any discomfort in your lower back or the sacroiliac joint area while doing this exercise, try bending your right knee and placing your right foot on the floor. If you still have discomfort, then don't do this exercise and go onto the next.

Relax your shoulders, relax your neck, and relax your facial muscles. Take 5–10 long slow deep breaths. Remember to breathe in through your nose and out through your nose, letting your belly expand as you inhale and release as you exhale.

COMING OUT OF THE POSTURE: On your last breath, slowly flex your knee. Release your belt and lower your left leg/foot to the floor.

BENEFITS: This posture is a great stretch for the lower back. It brings flexibility to the hips and stretches the hamstrings — which often go hand and hand with lower back issues.

Tight hamstrings and tight lower back muscles

are directly related to low back problems.

"Reclining hamstring stretch" is a great posture

for stretching both areas while giving gentle traction

to the lumbar area of your spine.

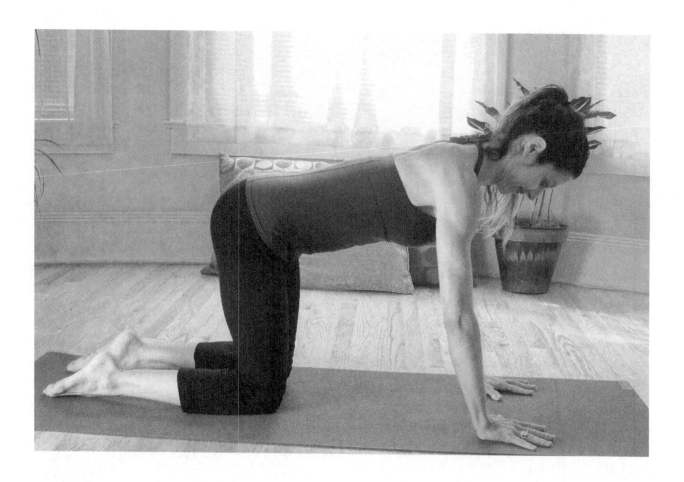

Table position

COMING INTO THE POSTURE: Position yourself on your hands and knees. You want to have your arms directly under your shoulders and your knees directly under your hips. Spread your fingers wide and make sure your middle finger is pointing straight ahead. Keep your head, neck, and spine in one line. You are now in table position.

From table position, slowly move your torso forward a little and then back a little. Forward a little and back a little. Increase the length of movement a little more each time so that your torso moves a little further past your hands and further past your knees when you go backwards. Be sure to move slowly — feel what is happing in your body. Repeat this back and forth movement for a total of 6–8 times.

COMING OUT OF THE POSTURE: After performing this movement 6–8 times, you can release this posture by sitting back on your heels and resting (if you find it difficult to rest on your heels, place a small pillow or rolled blanket between your buttocks and heels).

BENEFITS: This movement gently stretches the lower back and brings flexibility to your hips.

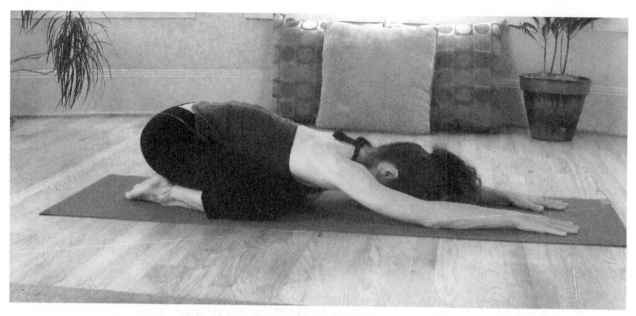

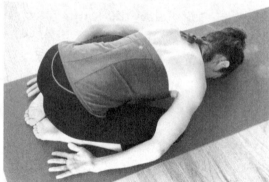

Child with arms along
the sides of the shins.

BENEFITS: Child's pose puts the hips into a neutral position, which allows the spine and muscles along the spine to stretch and relax. Child's pose also improves flexibility in the hips. It aids digestion, and is very soothing to the nervous system, making it great for reducing anxiety and promoting relaxation.

Child pose

GOING INTO THE POSTURE: You will begin by returning to the table position resting on your hands and knees. Take your knees a little wider than your hips and bring your big toes towards each other. Begin to sit back on to your heels, taking your hips towards your calves (if you have trouble sitting back, place a folded blanket or a pillow between your hips and calves).

Bring your chest towards your thighs and your head towards the floor. Extend your arms out in front of you or take them alongside of your shins with the palms facing up. Experiment with both versions and see which feels best to you.

If your head does not comfortably touch the floor, place a folded blanket under your head. You could also use one or two small pillows, a yoga block, or even your hands to support your head. In any case,

be sure not to force your forehead to the ground.

If you have any sensitivity on the outsides of your knees, you can put a blanket under your knees.

Take a moment and set up child's pose in a way that feels best. It is essential that this pose feel comfortable to you.

Once in child's pose, begin to breathe deeply in through your nose and out through your nose. Let your belly expand on the inhale; as you exhale, draw your belly button towards your spine. Continue to take a few more deep breaths here.

COMING OUT OF THE POSTURE: On your next inhalation, slowly lift your torso up. Rest your hips on your calves or simply come into a seated position on the floor.

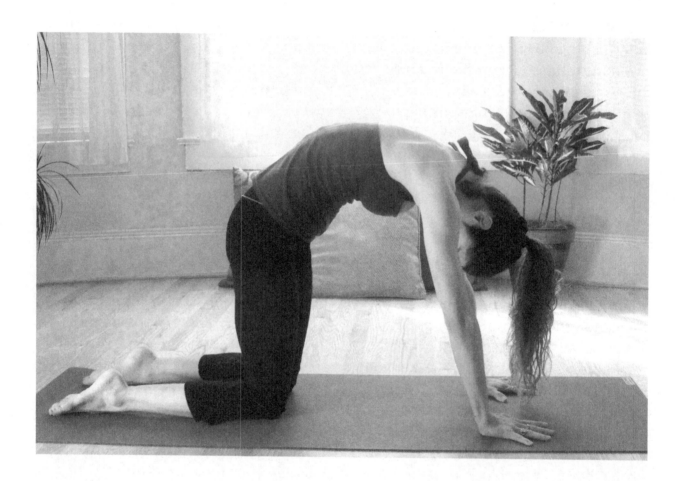

Cat tuck

GOING INTO THE POSTURE: Return to table position (resting on your hands and knees). Take a minute to make sure your arms are directly under your shoulders and your knees right under your hips.

Take in a deep breath and as you exhale, bring your head and hips towards each other, moving your belly button towards your spine. Press your hands into the ground and lift your shoulder blades towards the ceiling. Be sure to keep your arms straight. Hold for a second or two and then release. Inhale and drop your back to the starting position. Imagine a cat arching its back — this is what you want to look like.

Repeat this 3 more times on your own — going nice and slow — feel what is happening in your spine.

COMING OUT OF THE POSTURE: On your final inhalation, come back into a neutral table position, and then you can sit back on your heels and relax.

BENEFITS: Cat tuck pose puts your hips into a neutral posture and allows the muscles and facet joints of your low back to stretch in a controlled manner, which helps to increase flexibility along the spine. This posture also helps to stretch the entire spine as well as the shoulders and helps tone the abdominals. Cat tuck also helps to hydrate the vertebral discs, keeping them plump and functioning well.

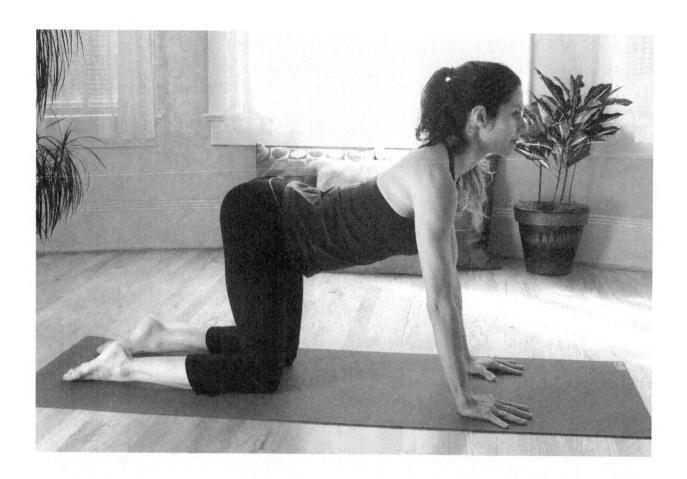

Dog tilt

GOING INTO THE POSTURE: Return to table posture. As you inhale turn your tailbone up towards the sky, rolling your hips over the tops of your thighs. Let your belly move towards the floor and lift your head and chest. Be careful not to compress the back of your neck. Keep your arms straight. Hold for a second or two. As you exhale, release and come back to table position.

Repeat dog tilt 4 more times. Go nice and slow — feel what is happening in your spine.

COMING OUT OF THE POSTURE: On your final inhalation, come back into a neutral table position, and then you can sit back on your heels and relax.

BENEFITS: Dog tilt enhances flexibility in the hips, lower back and mid back, and opens up the front of the spine. Dog tilt also helps to hydrate the vertebral discs, keeping them plump and functioning well.

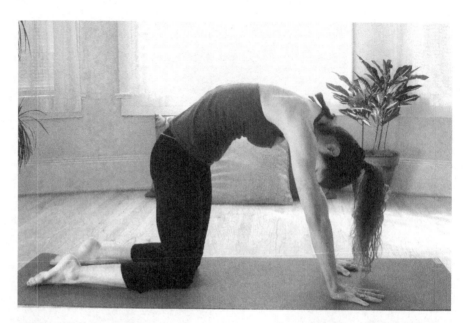

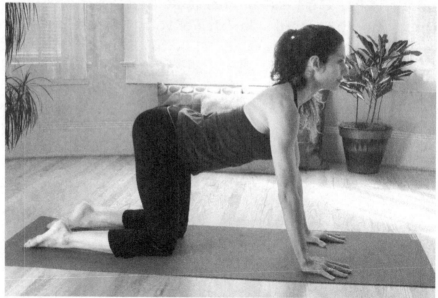

Cat tuck and dog tilt

Now we are going to combine the last two movements into one called cat tuck and dog tilt.

GOING INTO THE POSTURE: Starting in table position, take in a deep breath. As you exhale, bring your head and hips towards each other, moving your belly button towards your spine, arching your back like a cat. Hold for a second or two and then release.

As you inhale turn your tailbone up towards the sky, rolling your hips over the tops of your thighs. Let your belly move towards the floor and lift your head and chest. Be careful not to compress your neck. Hold for a second or two.

Now repeat this entire sequence of cat tuck and dog tilt three more times. Be sure to coordinate the movements with your breath. Go very slow, trying to feel each vertebrae as you go.

COMING OUT OF THE POSTURE: On your final inhalation, come back to a neutral table opposition, and you can sit back on your heels and relax.

BENEFITS: There are many benefits from practicing cat tuck and dog tilt. These include the stretching and strengthening of the lower back muscles, hip joints, and shoulders. The gentle slow movement introduces motion to the facet joints. Additionally, the discs between your vertebrae are being squeezed and soaked, which means that they are absorbing fluid which helps stop them from drying out. Your abdominal muscles are being engaged, and you are pumping cerebral spinal fluid to your brain, which is going to help you feel good, too!

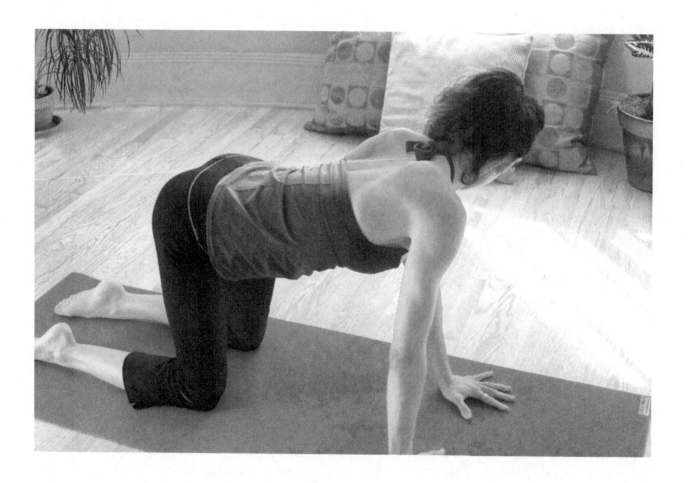

Doggy wag

GOING INTO THE POSTURE: Return to table posture. Make sure your arms are directly under your shoulders and your knees are directly under your hips, keeping your head, neck, and spine in one line.

Take in a deep breath. As you exhale slowly turn your head to the right, working to bring your right hip and the right side of your head towards each other — kind of like making the letter C with your torso. You want to move your hip towards the side of the head that is turning and not away from it.

As you inhale and slowly bring your head back to center, exhale and turn your head to the left, bringing the left side of your head and left hip towards each other.

Inhale and slowly bring your head back to center. Exhale and do the right side again — go slowly from side to side, working with your breath.

Exhale to the sides and inhale back to center. Repeat a total of 5–10 times.

COMING OUT OF THE POSTURE: On your final inhalation, you can sit back on your heels and relax.

BENEFITS: Doggy wag brings flexibility to the entire spine, brings fluid to the vertebral discs which helps keep them functioning properly, and also strengthens and stretches the abdominal muscles on the side of the body known as the obliques.

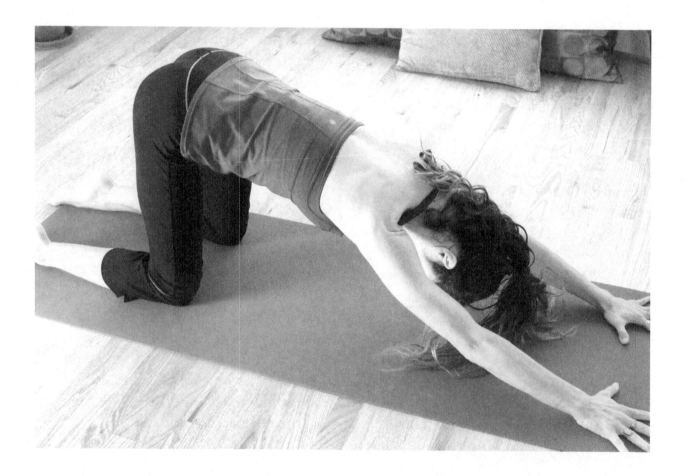

½ dog

GOING INTO THE POSTURE:
Return to table position with your arms under your shoulders and your knees directly under your hips. Begin to walk your hands forward until torso and arms are approximately 45 degrees to the floor. Keep your ears in line with your arms and your hips directly over your knees.

Make sure you are not pressing down on your shoulders. If this posture hurts your shoulders, then skip this posture and go on to the next. If you have sensitivity on the outside of your knees, placing a folded blanket under your knees will make this more comfortable for you. Take five slow deep breaths.

COMING OUT OF THE POSTURE: Inhale and walk your hands back towards your knees.

BENEFITS: ½ dog pose is a great stretch for your entire back as well as your shoulders and arms.

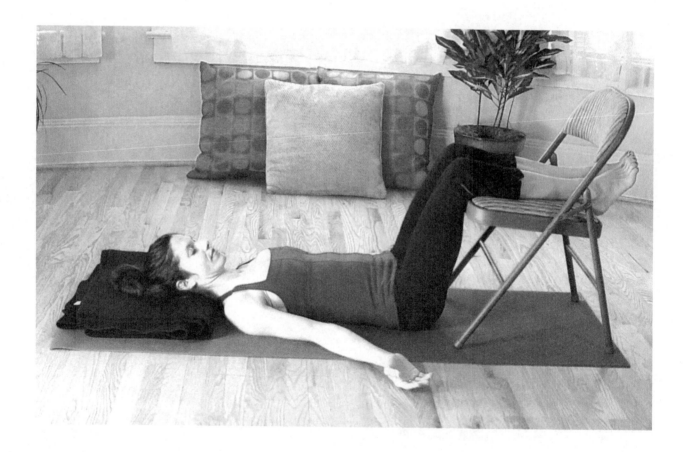

Legs on chair

Note: This is the last posture in the acute phase practice.

GOING INTO THE POSTURE: (You will need a chair to perform this posture and may also want to have a blanket or two nearby before you begin). Position a chair in front of you. Lie on your back and place your calves on the chair seat.

If you are a little on the shorter side, you will find it more comfortable to build up the floor by putting a folded blanket or two under your hips, back, and head. If you are on the taller side, you will find it more comfortable to put a folded blanket on the chair seat.

You will also want a folded blanket under your head as this is the best position for supporting your neck and for relaxing. You want to have your chin dropped slightly towards your chest.

Now, let your calves rest into the chair and your hips rest into the floor.

You can put your hands on your stomach or take them out to 45 degrees from your body with your palms up. Let your eyes close and your breath deepen. Rest here for 5–10 minutes.

BENEFITS: This posture is great for releasing the lower back, relieving lower back pain, improving circulation, balancing your energy, and is deeply relaxing for most people.

COMING OUT OF THE POSTURE: Let your breath deepen. Wiggle your fingers, wiggle your toes, and gently move your head from side to side. On your next exhalation, bring your knees into your chest and roll onto your right side into a fetal position.

Be there for a moment. Now, using your right and left hands slowly press up to a seated position.

THIS CONCLUDES THE YOGA PRACTICE FOR THE ACUTE PHASE OF LOW BACK PROBLEMS.

For optimal results in relieving lower back issues, we recommend that you practice this first section twice a day for 2–4 weeks

It is not uncommon for some people to experience a little stiffness or muscle soreness after the first or second day of this practice. If this is the case for you, we recommend that you apply ice or moist heat to the affected area as described in the first aid section of this book.

The next section focuses on building strength and flexibility in your lower back. Remember to always practice the postures from the acute sequence before doing this sequence as they prepare you for this second part.

Chapter Six

Yoga for Flexibility and Strength

This is the second part of our program, which focuses on building strength and flexibility in your back. This section should only be practiced after you have been practicing the first section for a minimum of 2–4 weeks and there is little or no back pain. Resist the urge to do this section until you are feeling little or no pain in your back. The exception to this is only if you have a healthy back to begin with, and you are using this program as preventative maintenance.

IMPORTANT: *Always do the postures in the first section to warm up before practicing these postures. Be sure to follow the sequence of postures provided. This will assure that you get the most out of your practice while staying safe. The exception to this is legs on chair pose which should be done at the end of your entire practice. Be sure to read through the postures before practicing them. Remember, if there is pain or discomfort at any time, stop, and do not do that posture.*

From table position, start by extending your leg back, coming onto the ball of your foot. Then stretch through your heel.

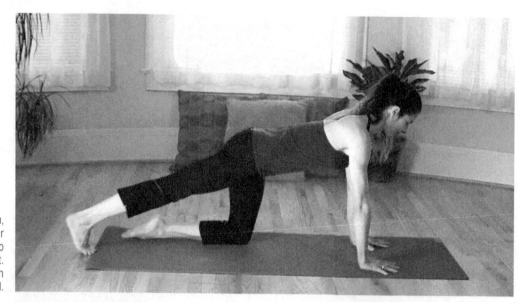

This is the final position. Optionally, you have both hands on the ground which will make this easier.

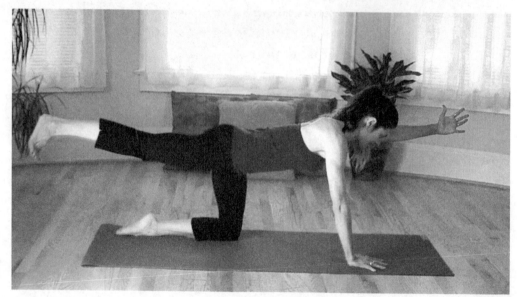

Cat balance

GOING INTO THE POSTURE:
Come into table position with your arms directly under your shoulders, your knees directly under your hips and your head, neck and spine in one line. Extend your right leg directly back behind you bringing toes onto floor and stretch into your heel.

Next, lift right leg to hip height and stretch through both heel and ball of foot. If you have your balance and want a little more challenge, then extend your left arm from your shoulder with the palm facing towards your center line.

Move your belly button towards your spine, reach through the right foot and reach through the fingertips of your left hand, making your body long. Hold for 5 breaths.

COMING OUT OF THE POSTURE: Bring your left hand to the floor and your right knee down. Now, do the other side. Extend your left leg directly back behind you bringing toes onto the floor. Stretch into your heel. Lift your left leg to hip height and stretch through both heel and ball of foot. If you want more challenge, extend your right arm from your shoulder with palm facing center line.

Move your belly button towards your spine, reach through the left foot and also reach out through the fingertips of your right hand, making your body long. Hold for 5 breaths. To release, bring your left hand to the floor and your right knee down.

BENEFITS: This posture is great for releasing your sacroiliac (SI) joints, stretching your lower back, and building strength through your abdomen as well as stretching your arms and shoulders. If you are experiencing any pain in your lower back or SI joint area while performing this posture, then skip this posture and go on to the next.

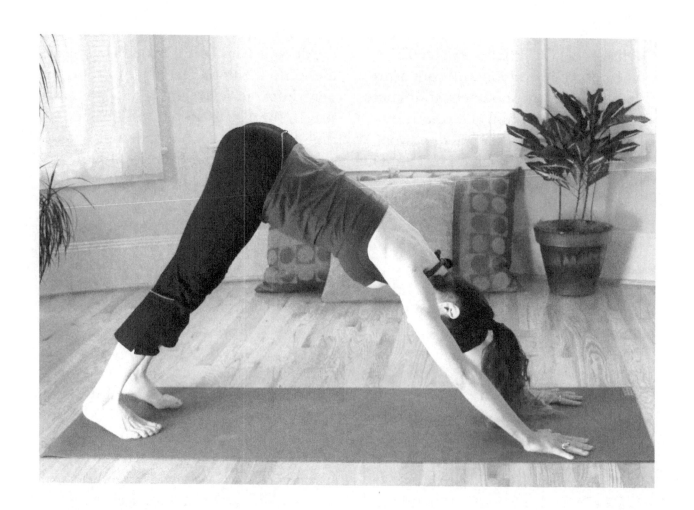

Downward facing dog pose

We are going to offer you two different versions of this posture. The first is downward facing dog pose on the floor, and the second is downward facing dog pose on a chair which should be used if you have super tight hamstrings, a tight lower back, or very tight shoulders.

DOWNWARD FACING DOG POSE (FIRST VERSION)

GOING INTO THE POSTURE:

Begin by coming into table position with arms under your shoulders and knees under your hips. Walk your hands forward about 8", so your arms are in front of your shoulders. Spread your fingers wide and make sure that your middle fingers are pointing straight ahead.

Next, as you exhale, press your hands and lift your hips high into the air, coming up on your toes. Press your hands and take your hips higher. Then, from the height of your hips, stretch your heels towards the floor. Your heels may or may not touch the floor — either way is fine.

Look back at your feet — they should be hip width apart. If you have tight hamstrings take your feet wider, closer to the sides of your yoga mat. This will make the posture a little easier for you.

Now, make sure your ears are between your arms and bring your awareness back to your hands and press into them, lengthening through your arms, lengthening through the sides of your torso, take your belly button towards your spine, and take your hips back more.

Press your thigh bones back towards your hamstrings and stretch into your heels.

Once you are in dog pose, take 5–10 long slow breaths. If you are new to yoga, this posture might feel a little challenging at first, so feel free to come out of the posture when you feel you need to. Rest for a moment, and then go back into the posture. Strength will come quick with practice.

COMING OUT OF THE POSTURE: Release onto your knees and rest in child's pose for a few breaths.

BENEFITS: Downward facing dog pose offers many benefits including: stretching the entire spine, stretching and building strength in the arms, shoulders and legs, and brings flexibility to the hips. In this posture, your head is lower than your heart, so it helps to bring circulation to your head area.

ALTERNATIVES:

If this posture is hurting your arms or shoulders, or you have trouble straightening your legs, even after taking them wider, then come down and perform the version of this posture on the chair, which follows next.

Also, if downward facing dog pose hurts your wrists in any way, then come down and roll up the front of your mat. Place the rolled mat area under the heel of your hand and your fingers on the floor. Using the rolled mat in this way will change the position of your wrist and works well for many people — however, if you are still experiencing discomfort in your wrists, then come out of this posture and practice dog pose on the chair.

Downward facing dog pose offers many

benefits including: stretching the entire spine, stretching

and building strength in the arms, shoulders and legs,

and brings flexibility to the hips. In this posture, your head is lower than

your heart, so it helps to bring circulation to your head area.

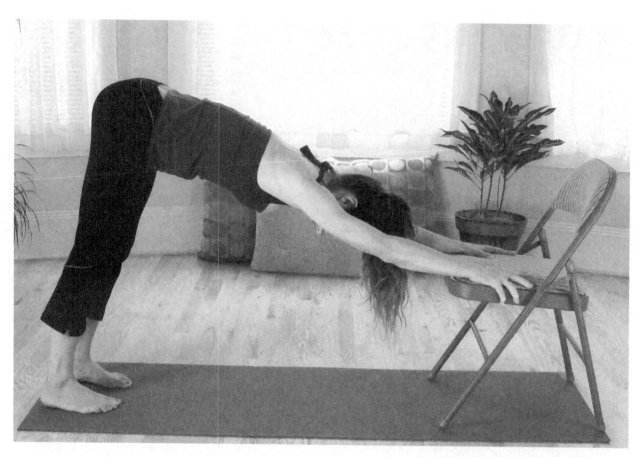

Make sure you walk your feet to the chair to come out of the posture.

Downward facing dog pose on the chair

Even if you were fine doing downward facing dog pose on the floor, you can also add this version as it has many benefits as well.

GOING INTO THE POSTURE:
Begin by placing a folding chair or armless chair with the back of the chair against the wall and on a yoga mat as shown.

Step up to the chair and face it. Place the palms of your hands on the front of the chair seat and begin to walk your legs back until they are a little behind your hips.

Your arms should be fully extended and your legs about hip width apart. If you have tight hamstrings or calves, then take your feet a little wider apart.

Make sure your feet are pointing straight ahead and that your ears are in line with your arms.

Now lengthen through your arms, lengthen through your torso, lengthen through the sides of your waist, move your belly button towards your spine, and take your hips back a little more.

Take 5 slow deep breaths here. This posture is a great stretch for the lower back, brings flexibility to the hips, stretches the hamstrings and calves, and stretches the shoulders and arms.

COMING OUT OF THE POSTURE: Walk your feet towards the chair and come to standing.

Note: Remember if downward facing dog pose feels too strenuous or uncomfortable to you, then you can try this version on the chair. And if this feels like too much, you can always practice ½ dog pose as described in the first section on yoga postures.

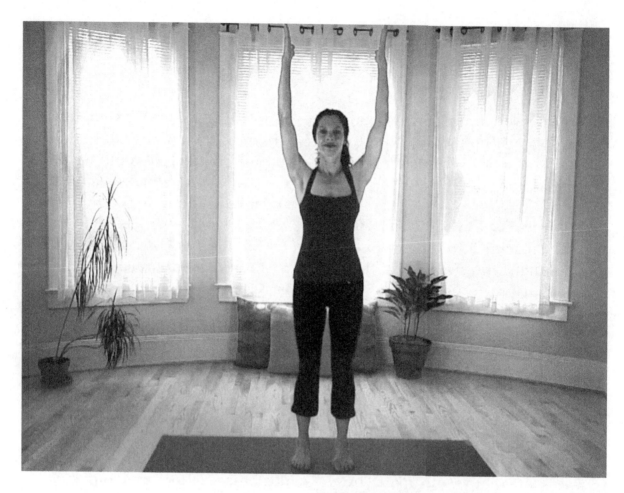

BENEFITS: The benefits of Tadasana include bringing your body into proper alignment, strengthening your legs, lengthening your spine, and stretching your shoulders and arms.

Tadasana / mountain pose

GOING INTO THE POSTURES:
Begin by standing with your legs directly under your hips and your feet pointing straight ahead. Make sure your torso is directly over your hips. Lift your toes and spread them wide. Keeping your toes spread, place them back on the floor. Balance evenly across the balls of your feet and your heels.

Pull up on your knees and thighs firming your thighs, and from the firmness of your thighs lift the sides of your waist and the sides of your chest. Lift your collar bones and draw your shoulder blades down your back and into your torso.

Keep your head, neck, and spine in one line, and make sure your jaw is parallel to the floor. Lengthen through your neck and out through the crown of your head. Take a couple of deep breaths here.

Now, take your arms out to the sides to shoulder height with your palms facing up completely. Stretch from the center of your chest into your fingertips. Take a couple of breaths.

Next, take your long arms up over head with palms facing each other and your arms in line with your shoulders. If you have tight shoulders, let your arms come forward a little bit.

Once again press into your feet, pull up on your knees and thighs, lift the sides of your waist, lift the sides of your chest, and lengthen through your arms and out through your fingertips. Take a few more deep breaths.

COMING OUT OF THE POSTURE: Exhale and lower your arms and notice how you feel.

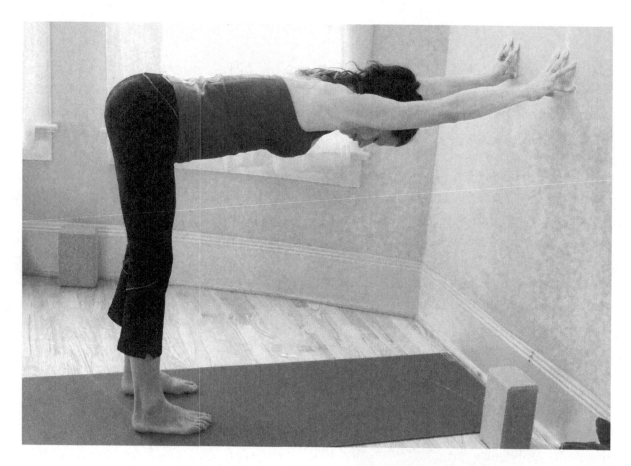

BENEFITS: Wall hang is great for stretching the spine, releasing the lower back, opening the shoulders, and stretching the hamstrings and calves.

Wall hang

GOING INTO THE POSTURE:
Place a yoga mat perpendicular to a wall or closed door as shown in the photo. Stand about 6" in front of the wall or door. Bring your fingertips onto the wall at mid-chest level. If you have any issues in your fingers or hands that prevent you from coming onto your fingertips, you can place your palms on the wall.

Keeping your finger tips or palms on the wall, begin to walk your feet back until your torso is more or less parallel to the floor. Make sure your legs are directly under your hips and your feet are pointing straight ahead. Ideally you want your arms and shoulders to be in one line.

If you have tight shoulders, then take your hands several inches higher up the wall. On the other hand, if you have very flexible shoulders make sure that you are not pressing them down but keep them in line with your arms.

Next, lengthen through your arms, lengthen through the sides of your torso, move your belly button towards your spine, and take your hips back a little more. Take a few long slow breaths.

Now, take the right side of your hips back a little more, then take the left side back a little more. Now, take both hips back a little more. Take a few more breaths.

Note: If there is any discomfort when taking one side of the hips back or the other, then do not do this variation and keep your hips straight.

COMING OUT OF THE POSTURE: On your next inhale, walk your feet towards your hands and come up.

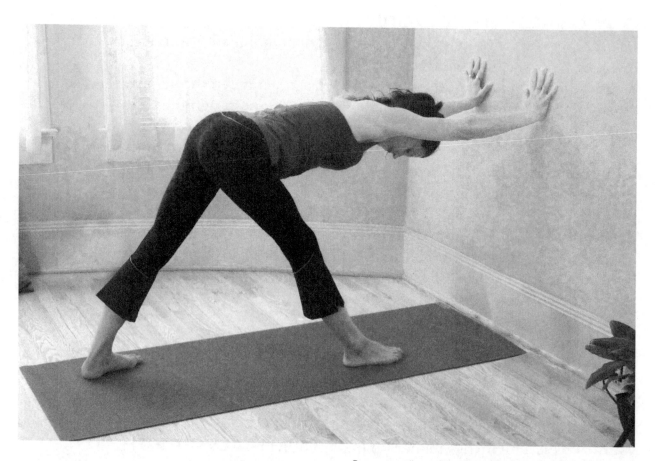

Be sure to walk your back foot alongside the front foot when coming
out of the posture, so you don't stress your lower back.

Parsvottanasana

The next posture is like wall hang only with one leg forward and one leg back.

GOING INTO THE POSTURE:

Stand approximately 12 inches away from a wall with your toes pointing straight ahead towards the wall. Then, bring your finger tips or palms to the wall like you did in wall hang, at about mid chest level.

Next, step your left foot back about the length of one of your legs, and turn your left foot out at 60 degrees as shown in the photo.

You want to end up with your torso almost parallel to the floor. If you have tight shoulders, take your hands several inches higher. Square your hips, bringing them in line with each other and approximately equidistant to the floor.

This posture can be a big stretch in the back of the legs, so make sure you are not feeling any stretch in the back of your knees — if you do, then bend your front knee slightly.

Now, lengthen through your arms, lengthen through the sides of your torso, take your belly button towards your spine, and take your hips back more.

COMING OUT OF THE POSTURE:

Take your left back foot towards your front foot and come up, and then do the other side. Take your right foot back about a leg's length and turn your right foot out at 60%. Lengthen through your arms, lengthen through the sides of your torso, take your belly button towards your spine, and take your hips back more. Take a few more deep breaths here, and then come out of the posture by moving the back foot alongside of the front.

BENEFITS: The benefits of Parsvottanasana include stretching the legs, hips, entire spine, shoulders, and arms.

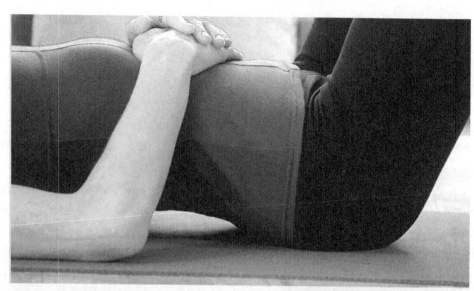

The 6 o'clock position, pressing your tailbone into the floor.

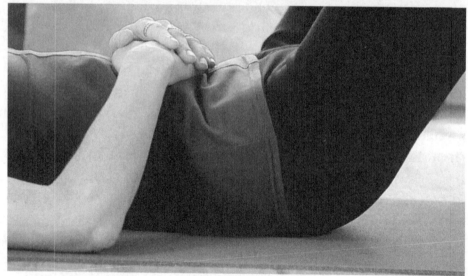

The 12 o'clock position, pressing the top of the sacrum into the floor.

Transition to floor

The next few postures are going to be done on the floor, so take a moment now to transition onto your back. You will need a yoga block or blanket for one of the poses, so take a moment to get that now.

Pelvic clocks

GOING INTO THE POSTURE:
Come onto your back with your knees bent and feet on the floor. Make sure your knees are in line with your hips. Bring your awareness to your tailbone, rock your hips forward and press your tailbone into the floor — this is the 6:00 o'clock position.

Now rock your hips back, releasing your tailbone from the floor and press the top of your sacrum towards the ground. This is the 12:00 o'clock position.

Go back to pressing your tailbone — the 6 o'clock position. And then rock back to the 12 o'clock position — pressing your sacrum towards the floor. Go back and forth a few times.

Now press your right hip into the ground — this is the 3 o'clock position. Release and press the left hip into the floor — this is the 9 o'clock position. Go back and forth a few times.

Next bring your attention to the 12 o'clock position and press down at the sacrum, then slowly pressing down at the 1 o'clock position, then slowly pressing

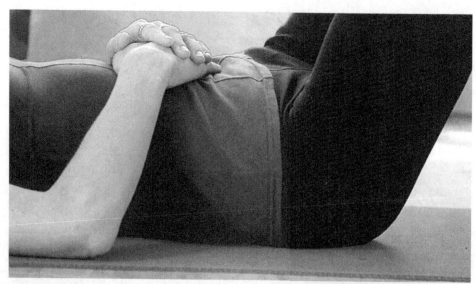

The 3 o'clock position, pressing the right hip into the floor.

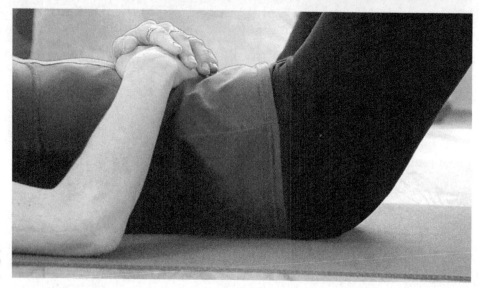

The 9 o'clock position, pressing the left hip into the floor.

down at the 2:00 o'clock position. Then slowly pressing down at the 3:00 o'clock position, then slowly pressing down at the 4:00 o'clock position. Then slowly pressing down at the 5:00 o'clock position. Then slowly pressing down at the 6::00 o'clock position. Then slowly pressing down at 7:00, 8:00, 9:00, 10:00, 11:00 and 12:00 o'clock positions.

Now you'll go backwards, pressing the 11:00 o'clock position to the floor, then the 10, 9, 8, 7, 6, etc. working your way back to 12:00 o'clock, the starting position.

BENEFITS: The benefits of performing pelvic clocks include strengthening the muscles of the lower abdomen and the entire pelvic area, which has a stabilizing effect. Pelvic clocks also help to bring strength and flexibility to the lower back and hip joints.

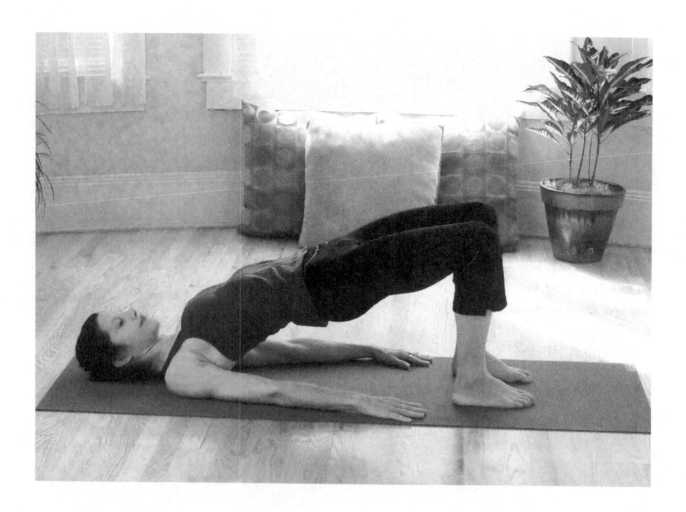

Bridge pose

GOING INTO THE POSTURE:
Continuing on your back, keep your knees bent and your feet on the floor. Make sure your knees are in line with your hips and bring your shins under your knees as much as possible. Your toes should be pointing in slightly and heels out slightly.

Take your arms alongside of your torso with your palms facing down towards the floor. As you inhale, slowly lift your hips off the floor, pause for a second or two, and then as you exhale slowly lower your hips towards the floor.

Again, inhale, slowly lift your hips off the floor, pause for a second or two, and then as you exhale slowly lower your hips towards the floor. Repeat this movement for a total of 5–10 times. On the last repetition, keep your hips up off the ground for a slow count of 10.

COMING OUT OF THE POSTURE: To come out of bridge pose, simply bring your hips to the floor and take a couple breaths before moving onto the next posture.

BENEFITS: Bridge pose is great for building strength and flexibility in your back, helps to tone the abdominals, builds strength in the hamstrings, and stretches the psoas and quadriceps muscles as well as the entire groin area.

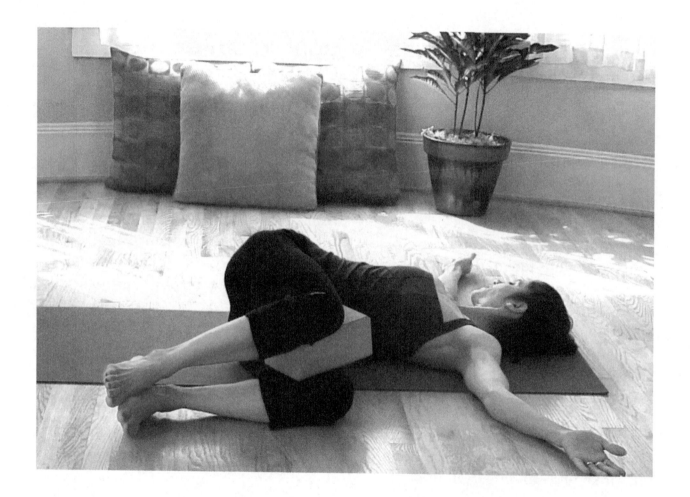

Knee down twist with block

Note: For this posture, you will need a yoga block or blanket.

COMING INTO THE POSTURE:

Start by laying on your back with your knees bent — just like you did in bridge pose. Place your yoga block between your knees, or you can also use a blanket which has been folded a few times. The block or blanket between your knees will help you from overstretching your lower back.

Extend your arms out to your sides at shoulder height with palms facing up. Next, lift your hips and scoot them to the right a little bit and set them back on the floor. Take your knees into towards your chest and then up and over towards the left side of your body. Allow your feet to come to the floor.

Look back towards your right hand. Take a total of 5–10 long slow deep breaths here.

Next, lift your knees up to center and put your feet on the ground, and you will do the other side. Lift your hips a little and scoot them a little to the left of center. Take your knees in towards your chest and then up and over towards the right side of your body. Allow your feet to come to the floor. Look back towards your left hand. Take 5–10 long slow deep breaths.

COMING OUT OF THE POSTURE:

To come out of the posture, lift your knees up to center, put your feet on the ground, and release your block or blanket. Roll to your right side and come up to a seated position.

BENEFITS:

The benefits of the knee down twists include stretching the muscles of the lower back, upper back, shoulders, and chest. Knee down twists also stretch the glutes and the piriformis muscles. The abdominal muscles also get stretched and toned and digestion is improved.

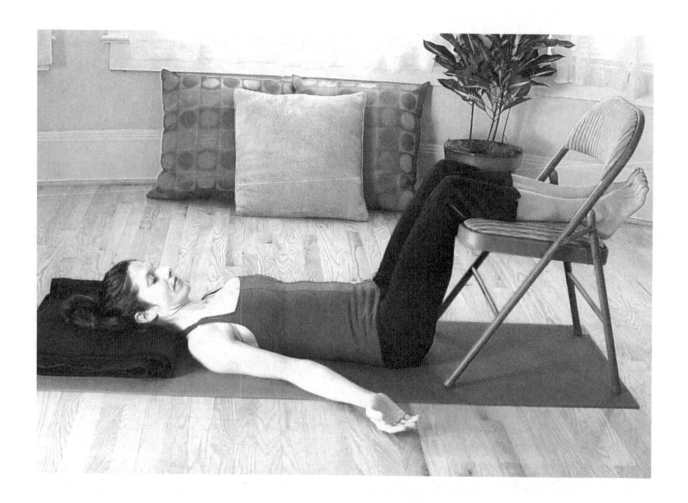

Legs on chair

The last posture in this sequence is legs on chair pose, which has been described in the first sequence; for convenience, we have provided it here again.

GOING INTO THE POSTURE:

(You will need a chair to perform this posture and may also want to have a blanket or two nearby before you begin). Position a chair in front of you. Lie on your back and place your calves on the chair seat.

If you are a little on the shorter side, you will find it more comfortable to build up the floor by putting a folded blanket or two under your hips, back, and head. If you are on the taller side, you will find it more comfortable to put a folded blanket on the chair seat.

You will also want a folded blanket under your head as this is the best position for supporting your neck and for relaxing.

You want to have your chin dropped slightly towards your chest.

Now, let your calves rest into the chair and your hips rest into the floor.

You can put your hands on your stomach or take them out to 45 degrees from your body with your palms up. Let your eyes close and your breath deepen. Rest here for 5–10 minutes.

BENEFITS: This posture is great for releasing the lower back, relieving lower back pain, improving circulation, balancing your energy, and is deeply relaxing for most people.

COMING OUT OF THE POSTURE: Let your breath deepen. Wiggle your fingers, wiggle your toes, and gently move your head from side to side. On your next exhalation, bring your knees into your chest and roll onto your right side into a fetal position.

The beautiful thing about yoga is that you can practice it just about anywhere at anytime. And you always have everything you need to practice with you.

Chapter Seven

First Aid for Your Lower Back

If you are experiencing acute lower back pain (pain from injuries occurring within 24–48 hours), then the following natural methods will help you reduce your level of pain.

First and foremost, the application of cryo or ice pack therapy has proven time and again to be one of the most effective ways to reduce low back pain following an acute or recent injury.

The application of ice therapy to an injured area reduces swelling, tissue, inflammation, muscle spasms, and pain. At the same time, the ice enhances the flow of nutrients into the area, aids in the removal of metabolites (waste products), increases strength, and promotes healing. To do this you must apply an ice pack to the painful area for a period of 24 to 48 hours as follows:

- For WOMEN/children the time limit is: 15 min. on, then 30 min. off

- For MEN the time limit is: 20 min. on, then 30 min. off

Remember…when using ice, never place the ice directly on your skin as it can burn the skin much like a frostbite injury. Always use a single layer of towel between the ice pack and skin.

You can also lay on the floor on your back with your knees bent and feet flat on the floor for 20 min. intervals. This will allow the low back muscle and facet joints to relax and stretch. A variation of this position is the legs on chair pose described in the last two chapters.

A word of a caution: If on a scale of 1–10, the pain in your lower back is an eight or greater, then avoid these postures and contact your doctor right away.

A method of reducing chronic low back pain **after 48 hours** is the use of moist heat. The advantage of moist heat is that it is more comfortable on the skin, and it can temporarily reduce muscle spasm in the surrounding tissue by increasing circulation to the damaged tissue. The increase in circulation also helps remove waste and toxins accumulating in the damaged tissue. As the muscle tissue and spasm subside and relax, more flexibility is gained and the healing process can accelerate.

Moist heat can be created by using a moist heating pad. These are available at most drug stores. You can also take a hand towel, get it wet, and wrap it around a hot water bottle or heated herbal bean bag.

- For WOMEN/children the time limit is: 15 mins. on, then 3 hrs. off

- For MEN the time limit is 20 mins. on, then 3 hrs. off

We highly recommend that you avoid dry heat.

To help you sleep and reduce muscle spasms in the lower back, we recommend that you lay on your side when in bed. Place a small pillow or folded towel between your knees. This will take the pressure off of your back (joints/disc) which should help relax the low back musculature. (Just a small side note… avoid laying on the sofa because it won't support your back properly.)

About the Authors

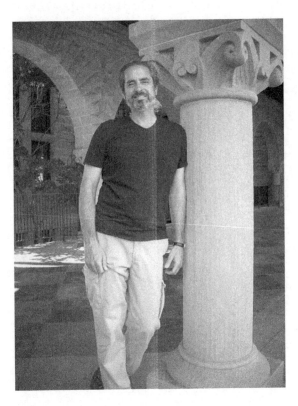

Howard VanEs, M.A., E-RYT 500 has been committed to wellness and fitness for over 28 years. He has a deep passion for helping people learn about the many ways they can improve the quality of their health and lives through mind/body methods.

For over 23 years, Howard has been a dedicated practitioner of hatha yoga and has been teaching yoga for the last 18 years in the Bay area of California. Howard has written many yoga related books, as well as numerous others focused on health and wellness.

His books include:

- *Beginning Yoga: A Practice Manual, Release Your Shoulders, Relax Your Neck. The best exercises for relieving shoulder tension and neck pain.*

- *ABS! 50 of the Best core exercises to strengthen, tone, and flatten your belly.*

- *Meditation: The Gift Inside. How to meditate to quiet your mind, find inner peace, and lasting happiness!*

- *Ageless Beauty & Timeless Strength: A woman's guide to building upper body strength without any special equipment.*

- *GERD & Acid Reflux Solutions. Your guide to prevention, treatment, cures, & relief!*

In addition to writing about and teaching yoga, Howard also leads yoga teacher trainings and wellness seminars and retreats worldwide.

Howard received a yoga teacher certification from Mt. Madonna Center in Watsonville, CA and has also received training from the advanced studies program at The Iyengar Institute of San Francisco. Howard also has an M.A. in counseling psychology.

His websites are www.letsdoyoga.com and www.booksonhealth.net.

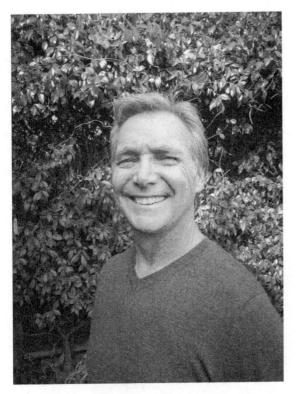

Dr. Richard Harvey, D.C.

For over 36 years Dr. Richard Harvey, D. C., C.C.S.P has been helping people heal through Chiropractic and other natural methods. He possesses an exquisite knowledge of the human body, how it functions, and what it takes to get and keep people healthy. He is certified in sports medicine and has worked with many high level athletes including Olympians, professional and college athletes as well as with many local sports teams, both as a coach and as well as providing ongoing care to team members.

Dr. Harvey graduated with honors from the renowned Palmer College of Chiropractic in Davenport, Iowa in 1976 and is certified as an Industrial Disability Examiner (I.D.E.). He and co-author Howard VanEs, have worked closely together to introduce yoga into his chirorpractic practice so that more patients as well as healthy members of the community can enjoy the many benefits of yoga for back care. Dr. Harvey has also teaches anatomy and physiology for the Letsdoyoga.com yoga teacher training program.

Connect with Dr. Harvey at www.harveychiropracticcenter.com

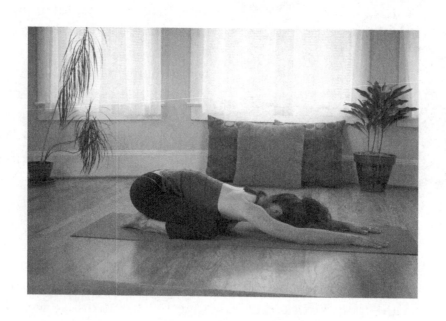

A special offer for readers of this book:

Get two FREE downloads: *Exercises You Can Do at Your Desk* and *Tips For Reducing Back And Repetitive Motion Injuries At Work*; especially good those who spend long hours on the computer!

Download them here: www.letsdoyoga.com/bonus

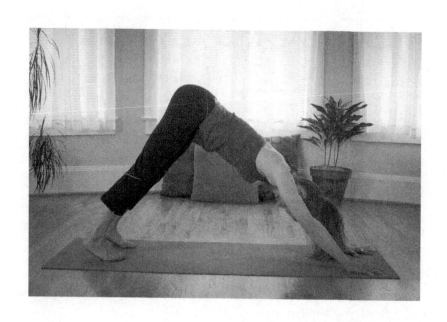

Additional publications of interest

All of the following books are available on Amazon.com and www.BooksOnHealth.net

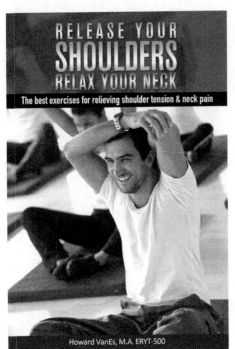

RELEASE YOUR SHOULDERS, RELAX YOUR NECK. THE BEST EXERCISES FOR RELIEVING SHOULDER TENSION AND NECK PAIN.

Do you suffer from shoulder pain or shoulder tension? How about neck pain?

Shoulder and neck pain can be very debilitating. Think about all the ways you use your shoulders and neck: whether it is working at a computer, driving, engaging in your favorite activities, turning your head, sleeping, or even picking up a fork to eat can be painful and difficult. The average shoulder injury causes a person to miss 28 days of work!

In "Release Your Shoulders, Relax Your Neck," you will discover:

- How to eliminate shoulder tension and neck pain with 53 highly effective shoulder and neck exercises.
- Photos of the exercises with easy to follow instructions.
- The main causes of shoulder and neck pain.
- Key prevention strategies to stop problems before they start, so you can have healthy shoulders and a pain free neck.
- Why computer users are at high risk for injury and what to do to significantly reduce your risk.
- How to speed healing of shoulder and neck injuries and get back into your favorite activities.
- Anatomy of the shoulder joints, how they move, and why they can get so tight.

This book is a must for people who work on computers, dental hygienists, hair stylists, athletes, and anyone who carries a lot of stress in his or her neck or shoulders.

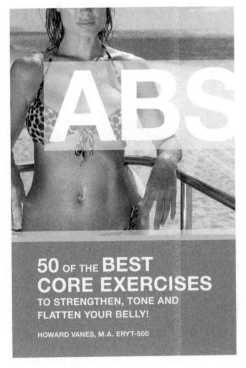

50 OF THE **BEST**
CORE EXERCISES
TO STRENGTHEN, TONE AND
FLATTEN YOUR BELLY!

HOWARD VANES, M.A. ERYT-500

ABS! 50 OF THE BEST CORE EXERCISES TO STRENGTHEN, TONE, AND FLATTEN YOUR BELLY.

Are you ready for a stronger, sleeker, slimmer belly? If so, then this book is for you!

Experience 50 of the very best ab and stomach exercises from Yoga, Pilates, and other fitness modalities. They have been carefully selected for their ability to produce quick results and are fun to do. ABS! goes well beyond old-fashioned crunches and sit-ups, so you can have an extremely effective abs workout.

Whether your belly is on the soft side or you're a high level athlete, you'll find a great variety of ab exercises that will target all four major groups of abdominal muscles, categorized as easy, moderate, and challenging – so it is great for all levels of fitness.

Abs! features 50 of the best exercises for your abs with photos and clear instructions, discussion of the many benefits of core exercises, an overview of anatomy and more!

MEDITATION: THE GIFT INSIDE. HOW TO MEDITATE TO QUIET YOUR MIND, FIND INNER PEACE, AND LASTING HAPPINESS

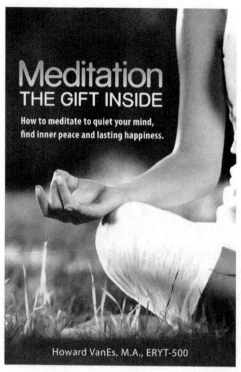

For thousands of years, people of faith, ascetics as well as everyday people have practiced meditation to quiet their minds, find inner peace, and connect with their spirit.

Whether you are looking for a book on meditation for beginners, or you are an experienced meditator wanting to renew your practice, you'll find "Meditation: The Gift Inside" connects you to the heart of the practice.

This meditation book covers:

- How to meditate like a yogi: experience the same meditation techniques that the deepest meditators use.
- Uncover the secrets to quiet your mind; have inner peace even when your outer world may be chaotic.
- Powerful methods to dramatically deepen your meditation.
- How to easily make meditation a part of your daily life and eliminate challenges that may prevent you from practicing regularly.
- Discover how modern scientific research is confirming what the ancient yogis knew about the extraordinary benefits of meditation including: sleeping better, reducing pain, improving mood, extending life, etc.

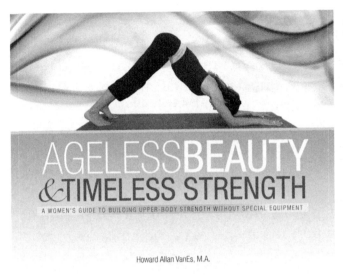

Howard Allan VanEs, M.A.

AGELESS BEAUTY & TIMELESS STRENGTH: A WOMAN'S GUIDE TO BUILDING UPPER BODY STRENGTH WITHOUT ANY SPECIAL EQUIPMENT

Discover one of the most important keys for longevity and why health experts are extremely excited about resistance training. Reverse osteoporosis: Strength training can stop the loss of bone AND increase bone mass by up to 9% within a year. Lose and maintain weight and stop yo-yo dieting. Reduce the risk of type 2 diabetes. Slow and prevent arthritis. Significantly reduce your risk of heart disease and high blood pressure. Could this be the fountain of youth? You decide!

Discover the life affirming benefits of fun body-weight only exercises to: Lose weight while becoming stronger and more toned! Sleep better and become healthier overall! Experience more self-confidence and look and feel your best! Have more energy and an enhanced sense of well-being!

Learn cutting edge nutrition secrets for maximizing strength and energy. Maximize your workouts to get the most benefits in the least amount of time. The book features fun, interesting, and challenging exercises for all levels.

BEGINNING YOGA: A PRACTICE MANUAL

Are you just getting started in yoga or an intermediate practitioner wanting to refine your practice? You will find "Beginning Yoga: A Practice Manual" will help you build a solid foundation and guide you through your home practice.

- Its large 8 ½ x 11 format makes it easy to use.
- A thoughtful balance of theory and practice are presented to provide you with a context as well as instruction for your practice.
- Fifty postures are shown with full page photos and clear step-by-step instructions for going into postures, coming out of postures, benefits of each posture, modifications, and cautions.
- Over 20 follow along practice sessions with words and pictures. Specific practices for energy, relaxation, and preventative back care. Lay flat book binding stays open for easy reference.

Chapters include: Intro to Yoga: history, philosophy, styles: Energy Body Basics: The Yogic Breath: Meditation 101 Pranayama (yogic breathing) Asanas (postures) and How to Practice Sequencing: Yoga Practices for Energy, Relaxation, etc.

NOTES

THE BACK PAIN CURE

NOTES